3 9085 00001468 4

S0-ARN-682

DIVA

UNLEASH YOUR FEMALE POWER

613.7045
'Wal

518517

Walsh, Terri
Diva

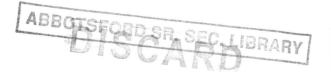

ABBOTSFORD SR. SEC. LIBRARY
DISCARD

Most Berkley Books are available at special quantity discounts for bulk purchases for sales promotions, premiums, fund-raising or educational use. Special books, or book excerpts, can also be created to fit specific needs.

For details, write Special Markets: The Berkley Publishing Group, 200 Madison Avenue, New York, New York 10016.

613.7045
Wal

518517

DIVA

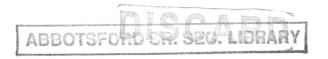

UNLEASH YOUR FEMALE POWER

Terri Walsh

with Catherine Whitney

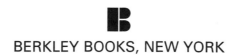

DISCARD

ABBOTSFORD SR. SEC. LIBRARY

B

BERKLEY BOOKS, NEW YORK

This book is an original publication of The Berkley Publishing Group.

DIVA

A Berkley Book / published by arrangement with the authors

PRINTING HISTORY
Berkley trade paperback edition / February 1998

All rights reserved.
Copyright © 1998 by Terri Walsh and Catherine Whitney.
Text design by Rhea Braunstein.
Cover design by Steve Ferlauto.
Photographs by Brad Guice.
This book may not be reproduced in whole or in part,
by mimeograph or any other means, without permission.
For information address: The Berkley Publishing Group,
a member of Penguin Putnam Inc.,
200 Madison Avenue, New York, New York 10016.

The Putnam Berkley World Wide Web site address is http://www.berkley.com

ISBN: 0-425-16158-7

BERKLEY®
Berkley Books are published by The Berkley Publishing Group,
a member of Penguin Putnam Inc.,
200 Madison Avenue, New York, New York 10016.
BERKLEY and the "B" design are trademarks belonging
to Berkley Publishing Corporation.

PRINTED IN THE UNITED STATES OF AMERICA
10 9 8 7 6 5 4 3 2 1

To the women of

Determination

Integrity

Vitality

Aspiration

who have come before us . . .

and all those yet to be

ACKNOWLEDGMENTS

My deepest gratitude to the many people who have given me
support, inspiration, belief, and motivation. In particular . . .

My mom and my brother. Thanks, I love you.
All of my friends who put up with me and allow me to put
up with them back.
Jane Dystel, my agent, who first saw the promise of DIVA.
Hillary Cige, my editor at Berkley, who believed in me.
Catherine Whitney, my coauthor, who guided me.
Paul Krafin, for his valuable input.
My students, who taught me about being a DIVA.
And all the women who were brave enough and committed
enough to share their hopes and dreams for this book.

CONTENTS

PART 1: The DIVA Spirit   I

1   My Story: Moving Through It   3
2   Your Body: Get Over It!   I I
3   DIVA: The Power System   2I
4   Everybody Starts As a Beginner   29

Part 2: The DIVA Work   4I

5   Strength, Balance, Energy . . . Life!   43
6   Determination   5I
7   Integrity   75
8   Vitality   99
9   Aspiration   I25

Part 3: The DIVA Life   I37

10   It's Your Life   I39
11   The Four Progressions of the DIVA System   I47
12   Food: DIVA's Best Friend   I77

DIVA Journal   I85

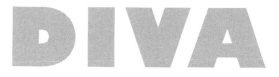

DIVA

UNLEASH YOUR FEMALE POWER

PART 1

THE DIVA SPIRIT

1

MY STORY: MOVING THROUGH IT

"Why don't you just kill me?"

I was hunched over in the middle of the room, half crying, half yelling. My face was throbbing where my stepfather had punched me, and something inside me had just cracked. For the first time since he had started physically and sexually abusing me eight years earlier, I stood up to him. But it wasn't bravery that compelled me. It was total and complete despair. I just didn't care anymore. I was fifteen years old, and I wanted to die.

My stepfather pulled back for a moment in surprise. I had never challenged him before, and my cry from the heart seemed to deflate him. I stumbled into my room and collapsed on my bed, but I didn't weep. I huddled there with my arms wrapped around my body and withdrew into a safe state of numbness where I felt nothing.

People who work with abused children will tell you that this type of disassociation is a common mode of survival. In some cases, the disassociative state becomes permanent, and the psychic injury never heals. At that moment, I was dangerously close to slipping off the edge.

On the day I confronted my stepfather, I guess my words struck a chord because he never touched me again. But it hardly mattered; the damage was already done. I had become weak, fearful, and empty—the product of a lifetime of physical and sexual abuse.

The feeling of weakness, the disassociation, developed with time. In the beginning, I fought tooth and nail. Even as a very young child, I knew it was wrong when my stepfather touched me. I kicked and yelled. I screamed, "I hate you!" and "You're a bad man!" My one victory was that he never achieved penetration, but in every other way, he won. Each time my stepfather hit me, I went deeper inside. Each time he touched me, I became colder and more unfeeling. Eventually, I stopped fighting. Since I didn't have the power to stop him, I simply gave up. Over time, failure became an easy place to be. I was used to feeling weak, to saying, "I can't stop this!" When you're abused as a child, you feel helpless and learn to withdraw. You try to protect yourself with frailty, with invisibility. I became a weak, frightened young woman who lived in shadows.

My stepfather got away with the abuse because my mother was constantly working to support us; he was always between jobs. I never told my mother what was happening. My stepfather convinced me she wouldn't believe me. He loved to taunt me with that: "You're nobody, and nobody will believe you."

But my mother had her own grievances with the cruel man who lived in our house, and their marriage finally ended. I still remember the day she kicked him out. As he left the house, he reached out and tried to kiss me. I turned my back and closed the door. A weight was lifted from my shoulders, but it took me many years to sort out my feelings. I'm still putting together the pieces of that puzzle now.

Today, at thirty-two, I can vividly remember the sensation of feeling that life held nothing for me. My stepfather tried to take away my identity, my strength. But in the end I was lucky. I'm telling this story for the first time because I know that before a woman can get fit, strong, and beautiful, she first has to know she exists—and push through the greatest barrier of all—the inability to believe in herself.

Climbing Out

How did I grow from that fragile, frightened young woman into the person I am today? That's the real story. I saved myself by getting strong—inside and out. And it didn't happen overnight. It happened one small step at a time.

By the time I was nineteen, I was drifting. All around me, I saw people my age forging ahead with energy and purpose. They had goals. They knew what they wanted. What was *my* purpose? I knew I was smart, but I had no idea what to do with myself. College bored me, so I dropped out after a couple of years and became a dabbler. I'd start one thing, give it up, and move on to the next. Nothing seemed to ignite any lasting passion in me.

Needing to work, I got a job as a locker room attendant at a Jack LaLanne fitness center. It was just a job for me, and a crummy one at that, collecting sweat-drenched towels and cleaning up after the members. I approached the work the same way I did everything else then: moving through the days without thinking much about it. But I began to find it impossible to remain remote in that environment. The pulsing energy of the place started to affect me. Soon I found myself eager to get to work. That was certainly a new experience! And I was reluctant to leave when my shift was over. I began hanging around, taking a few classes, experimenting with all the exotic and forbidding machines. Not only didn't I know what they were for, I could hardly manage any of the equipment. It was fun, but I felt pretty silly. Weak little me!

The gym's lifeguard, a muscular and athletic man who spent a lot of time in the weight room, noticed how hard I was working. He took a liking to me, and he seemed to recognize my potential. He saw something in me that I couldn't see in myself. He encouraged me to apply myself and become a skilled physical trainer. I started to work harder than I had ever worked in my life. Within a few months, at first almost imperceptibly, my body began to change. More importantly, however, my attitude began to change. Everything seemed different, better; this was a turning point for me.

Within a year, I was stronger and more confident than I had ever thought possible. But there were still facets of the old Terri. When the manager asked me to come on staff as an instructor and to teach an aerobics class, I literally turned around to see who he was talking to. *Me?* Was he kidding? No, he wasn't kidding. He gave me a chance. And so I began my career as a neophyte DIVA.

Teaching an aerobics class may not sound like a big deal, but it was a huge task for me. It was a direct challenge to everything I had initially thought about myself. What did it mean to be a great aerobics teacher, anyway? Nonstop energy? Did you have to be the best athlete in the class, the end-all and be-all? Where did the confidence to stand up there and lead a class come from? Could someone teach you how? The hardest part was believing I could do it. I was used to giving up and not seeing things through. I didn't trust myself enough to know that I'd hang in there. I thought people would walk into my class, take a look at me, and sneer, *"This* is supposed to be a teacher?" You see, although I had overcome many of the physical barriers, my mind was still holding me back. I didn't believe I had a right to happiness and success. In my heart, it didn't feel like *me*.

Maybe you've been there. People put you down for so long that you believe them. Your own good opinion isn't worth as much to you as their bad opinion. Amazing, isn't it? You begin to believe that you can't do things. You begin to believe that you don't deserve to feel good.

Belief can be a powerful force for both good and evil. When you can convince yourself that your opinions do matter and that you have the right to be happy and successful, then you've turned the negative belief around.

I'm not just talking about fitness. I'm talking about life. Because here's the secret I learned: Fitness and living your life are one and the same dynamic. The process of fitness is the process of learning to love your body, which means loving who you are. Physical strength and internal strength develop simultaneously. The qualities of determination, integrity, vitality, and aspiration that you bring to your workout begin to show up in your life.

The barriers that may have kept you from becoming fit and strong are the very barriers that seem to block you from everything else:

Do you have the *determination* to identify what it is that you really want?

Do you have the *integrity* to demand the best of yourself and to change what makes you unhappy?

Do you have the *vitality* to enter into almost any situation and make a positive difference?

Do you have the *aspiration* to strive for the very best you can achieve, to go after your dreams?

The DIVA System helps you define the qualities that delineate your true self, the person that you really are. Or at least who you were before everyone else started defining you by their terms. You don't have to live with an identity that was decided on by other people.

Explore your purest thoughts and feelings, and find out on your own. Always say to yourself: "It's *my* life. It's up to *me*." The result of this self-knowledge is a glorious sense of freedom and power. It's challenging, it's exhilarating, and it's worth the chance. Chance? What chance? The chance you won't stick with it, the chance you might feel silly, the chance you'll have aches and pains, the chance you'll hate it.

I discovered my own freedom and power through physical expression. I want to share that discovery with you. Come on, stick with me. Take a chance.

Speaking of Chances

When I began thinking about writing this book, I had to jump over another wall. The wall was called: What right does Terri have to give advice to other people? Who does she think she is?

Let's face it. There are hundreds of books that can tell you how to do a push-up, a squat, or an abdominal crunch. It isn't because I know something exceptionally clever about the dynamics of the body in motion or that I know exercises that nobody else has ever thought of before. I have something else I want to share with you.

What's important to me is to communicate a sense of power and self-worth to other women. It's so basic, isn't it? I find it remarkable that it isn't the essence of every fitness program designed specifically for women. I've read most of the fitness books lining the shelves: the ones written by professional bodybuilders, beautiful fashion models and actresses, and life-long fitness experts. I've done just about all of the exercises suggested and followed countless training regimens. I've longed to condense and assemble my own program in a way that engages women instead of making them feel inadequate.

Imagine what it would be like to read some of the fitness books out there if you are underweight or overweight or have never been physically active. Or what if—sin of sins—you weren't young anymore? Instead of feeling motivated, you'd read them and become depressed, more convinced than ever that you'd never be able to measure up.

I realize that you may not be in any of those categories. Many of the women who train with me and take my classes are fit and self-assured. Maybe you're like them, and you're reading this book because you want to perfect your skills. Even so, every woman can use an ally in fitness, not to mention a pep talk about self-esteem.

For me, self-esteem—feeling good about yourself—comes first. It's the primary goal. We'll get in shape sanely, safely, and realistically.

One step at a time.

2

YOUR BODY: GET OVER IT!

Ask any woman to describe her body. What will you hear? I know, because I've asked thousands of times. You'll hear:

I'm fat.
My legs are stubby.
My butt is flabby.
I'm too short.
I'm too skinny.
My stomach is soft.
My back is ugly.

And on and on and on. How often do you hear a woman, no matter how she looks, say, "My body looks great"? Not very often. Women hardly ever feel confident enough about their looks to say such things. You can be a model of fitness and still worry about how you look or how much you weigh or a little bulge here and there.

It really burns me how women are taught from an early age to be supercritical of the way their bodies look. And the self-

"Dating back to high school, I always had a negative impression of my body. I often thought, 'If I could just lose some weight from my thighs and behind, my life would be completely different.' I hated being so shallow, but it was difficult not to want some model or movie star's body, considering that was the ideal. Look at the women today. Cindy Crawford, Claudia Schiffer, Vendela; I mean, what's changed?"

Martha, 30

....

"I always felt I was too fat and my legs were ugly. As a child I was always told, 'You have such a pretty face. If only you lost some weight, you'd be so much cuter.' I've always wished I had almost anyone else's body except mine."

Jane, 28

....

"I know I'm deluded, but I've been comparing myself to anorexic, eighty-pound women my whole life. I'm still extremely critical of myself and see every ounce of weight I gain. Once during dinner my father said, 'Keep eating like that and your ass will be as wide as the back of a bus.' I just burst into tears."

Fran, 40

criticism is not related to being healthy, fit, and strong. It's about desperately wanting to conform to a cultural ideal. You rarely hear men complaining that they can't succeed because of the way they look. Powerful men come in all shapes and sizes. A far different message has been created for women.

Too many women have grossly warped pictures of their bodies. For example, Peggy, a lovely young woman in her twenties, told me, "Although I've always been thin, I'm short. My sister has very long legs—mine are stubby. Whenever I look in the mirror, I see a short, chubby person with thick legs. It's hard to see what other people see. I know my legs aren't that short or thick. They aren't willowy either, but they are shapely and muscular. I know that intellectually, but emotionally, I still see short, thick stubs!"

I ask you: Where does *that* come from? Well, one thing is for sure: These perceptions don't just suddenly erupt. You have to be taught that you don't measure up or that you should look a certain way. Women who have been taunted about their bodies—either because they were desirable or not—know just what I mean. I asked some women to be candid about their experiences. Their responses appear throughout the book, maybe you'll relate to them.

There are endless numbers of stories like these, tales of humiliation and embarrassment suffered because not all women are "perfect." That image of perfection is only a commercial and cultural myth anyway. It changes according to the whims of some mysterious group of fashion designers and Hollywood executives. And we buy into it. What a joke!

As I hear women express their unhappiness and regret at being unable to achieve some arbitrary vision of the perfect woman, I become more determined than ever to get this message across: Strength—from the inside out—equals beauty. It's fundamental. You can't feel and see your beauty until you feel and see your strength.

I'm not saying that strength is an easy concept to master at first. But the process of discovering how to gain strength can be a wonderful journey all in itself.

Get Real About Your Body

Recently, a new client of mine called me on the phone. She was very upset. In addition to her workouts with me, she had also been going to Weight Watchers. Her goal was to lose thirty pounds, and she had just returned from her weekly weigh-in.

"I didn't lose an ounce!" she wailed. "In fact, I *gained* half a pound."

I tried to console her by explaining the facts of body weight. "Don't worry," I said, "that's because you're gaining muscle. Muscle weighs more than fat."

There was a long silence on the other end of the phone. In a stunned whisper she finally said, "You mean I'm going to weigh *more* if I keep working out?"

"Maybe, but you'll look thinner and better toned," I said. "Your dress size will go down. In fact, you are already starting to get those results. You told me just yesterday that you loved the way your body was looking."

But that wasn't good enough. She couldn't deal with the idea that the number on the scale might not be what she thought it should be. She couldn't let go of some idealized weight and concentrate instead on how her body looked and felt. Discouraged by conflicting information and nagged by doubt, she decided to go for the numbers. She stopped exercising.

"Remember high school, that bastion of self-confidence? I was on the track team, and a boy that I had a secret crush on called me 'thunder thighs.' Thunder thighs? My quadriceps were overdeveloped. I had great legs. What a jerk! That one stupid thing has stayed with me for twenty years now."
Abby, 35

"When I started wearing training bras, my older stepbrother used to call me 'flatsy.' He and my dad used to make gross Band-Aid jokes all the time. It really got old fast, y'know? To top it off, the class clown in high school singled me out. This guy would follow me down the hallway barking, and he called me 'dog face' all the time. I don't even know how I stayed sane when I think about it."
Gloria, 31

"As a kid, I got bugged a lot because I was heavy. I also was very developed by the time I was twelve. I dreaded having to change for gym class in front of the other girls, and then be forced to try things I couldn't do—like gymnastics and rope climbing. I always left class feeling terrible. The other girls were so mean, joking about my clumsiness."
Mary, 38

"When I was in sixth grade, I was tall and overweight. I remember riding my bike past a group of kids in my neighborhood. They all chased after me, laughing and yelling out, 'Hey, Big Mama!'"

Elise, 27

This obsession with weight is epidemic among women. The very idea of getting on that scale and watching the numbers creep up makes their hair stand on end. I know women who feel simply fabulous—until they weigh themselves. Destroy the damn scales. Stop believing the hype. Normal weights based on height and age are a fiction manufactured by insurance conglomerates for their actuarial tables. They never take into account body types or the effect of exercise on your musculature and metabolism. How can some pencil pusher in an insurance company possibly determine what weight is best for you? Instead, try to imagine what it would feel like to judge your progress by how you feel and by how you look in your own eyes.

Here's what I see every day: A lot of women care more about the number on the scale than what that number may really represent. They see the ideal body as being thin but voluptuous in the right places, firm, but not too firm. Many women view their bodies as something to look at, not something that functions.

It's not too surprising. There is an enormous industry vying for women's attention. Food, clothing, and cosmetic companies prod women to eat this, wear that, and smear eyeshadow and skin cream on their faces while doing it.

I think we should just hold on for a second. Let's face facts. Women's bodies are fit for function as well as form. This isn't shocking new information, but I think we need to be reminded. All of us need to live, to work, and to play.

One of the ways to begin bringing it all together is by getting in touch with the key elements necessary for efficient function. One of those key elements is available to us at all times— our bodies.

I've designed a series of exercises that should make your

body feel integrated and unified with the DIVA spirit I hope to share with you. You owe it to yourself to fully inhabit your body—to feel comfortable in your own skin. You need to focus more on how you feel when you move than on how you look.

I know the fitness business is full of angles: big promises, hot-button issues, seductive advertising, and ploys. Recently, I was approached to do a magazine feature on fitness instructors. The editor welcomed me like I was a member of some elite team, then asked, "What's your gimmick?"

I honestly responded without a second thought. "I don't have a gimmick. I have a *life*."

DIVA is not a gimmick. It's a name I've attached to my promise that every woman can be satisfied living in her body. DIVA is my personal call-to-action statement—my call to movement.

THE FIVE FEARS AND THE FIVE VICTORIES

What can you look forward to? What does success really mean? What's been holding you back?

I find that many women approach the initial process of fitness training with a number of sometimes irrational fears. You have to make a leap of faith and simply take it one small step at a time. Usually, every fear you have will loom up immediately—and disappear just as quickly. Without fail, it only takes one session for my clients to identify their fears and slay them. Believe me, it's liberating. It's a real eye-opener for people. It isn't coincidental that the fears you face with me are probably the same fears that hold you back in every other important area of your life.

First is *the fear of success*. I know that sounds ridiculous, but it's the biggest fear I run across. When you make a commitment to be strong, you have to leave behind all of your previous misconceptions and say good-bye to your old, weak self-image: the safe friend, the hideout, the part of you that rewarded you for not standing up for yourself. You begin to accept the fact that you are strong and competent, and then you have to back it up. Once you say, "I can lift weights," or "I can run three miles," you have to be the person who can do that. You can't let yourself off the hook anymore.

The second fear is *the fear of looking stupid*. I know this one sounds frivolous, but I see it all the time, especially when people are just starting out. How can anyone become good at anything without making a mistake? Impossible. Amid the multitude of other messages women have pounded into them from birth, there is the one that insists that women have to look cool, calm, and possessed in every situation. No mistakes allowed. I know for an absolute fact that some women absolutely believe that they can get fit without ever breaking a sweat! There's also that horrible feeling of being hopelessly clumsy and contorted because you're just beginning and you haven't mastered all the moves. This happens even when you're working out alone—when you glance at yourself in the mirror and grimace at how silly you look. Well, there are a lot of human activities that look awkward and silly (like sex, for example), but if you really get into it, you forget how you look.

Third is *the fear of being strong*. This is simply being afraid that you'll lose your femininity, that you won't be appealing anymore, that you'll look muscular and masculine. Guess what? Women respond to strength training differently than men. It's the difference between being estrogen driven (female) and testosterone driven (male).

The best antidote to this fear of being strong is to look at female athletes who are very strong but manage to exude powerful feminine qualities. Katarina Witt, Jackie Joyner-Kersee, Lisa Leslie, and Gabrielle Reece are just a few in the burgeoning ranks of women who are exemplars of athletic grace and strength.

The fourth fear is *the fear of failure*. If you haven't used your body in this way before, you may not trust it. Perhaps you're afraid it won't hold up, that it will let you down. It's that feeling of panic you sometimes get when you have to lift something unusually heavy and you're not sure you can handle it; that second when you begin to jump over a mud puddle and you're worried you might not make it. Maybe you've started and dropped out of other exercise programs, and you're afraid that it's a cycle you can't break. There's only one way to conquer that fear. Confront it, accept it, and move on.

The fifth fear is *the fear of pain*. No one is in love with pain. You may think it's really going to hurt to stretch your muscles or move until you start breathing hard. It's all right; I understand. Sometimes it does. That's the pain that comes from being stagnant. I'm not interested in hurting you. I'm only interested in helping you.

So, take it easy. There's no reason to get carried away at first. You have to build up your tolerance and endurance slowly.

Of course, real pain isn't part of any responsible fitness program. If you try to do too much too soon, and a specific body part feels as though a ball peen hammer has been repeatedly smashed into it, that's the pain of injury. But the other pain you imagine has a different name; it isn't real pain, but discomfort. And why not? If you've never used your body like this before, you may not know what it should feel like to be so active. In the beginning, it may feel very uncomfortable and unnatural. Once your body adapts to the various movements, your initial discomfort is replaced by a feeling of power. You'll be shocked at how quickly you come to enjoy it. It becomes fun to challenge yourself, and it's a source of pride to gauge your progress.

When you overcome the five fears, you have the potential to experience what I call the five victories. These are:

- Confidence: the can-do attitude.
- Release of worry: the faith that this is going to happen. It's just a matter of going with the system and believing that the effort will be worth the result.
- Trust in your body: Your body is an amazing feat of advanced bioengineering. It won't fail you; it won't let you down.
- Proficiency: No one starts at the top. No one is a natural. You can master this.
- Owning the knowledge: Knowledge is not something outside of you. Once the knowledge is yours, it lives in you.

I'm always amazed by the lengths to which some women will go to avoid seeing their successes. I had a wonderful, fiercely devoted client recently, a woman who had made enormous strides while working with me. Her self-confidence had soared. It wasn't so much the pounds she had shed as the way she looked and moved. She was graceful, voluptuous, and strong all at once. In her late forties, she had worked like a demon for six months. In the process, she lost twelve pounds and several inches. When she ran into some old friends on a visit to her childhood home, they all remarked on how fabulous she looked. One woman went so far as to ask the name of my client's surgeon, implying that her rejuvenation was a brilliant job of surgical enhancement. My client didn't deny it. Instead, she told her friend that it wasn't just good genes that were responsible for her impressive looks. I was so angry when my client told me about it that I begged her to call her old friend and tell her how hard she had worked to look so great. Her beautifully toned body and her weight loss were her personal successes. She worked for it; it didn't just happen.

Learn to take credit for your achievements. Don't be afraid to stand up and say, "I worked for this."

Being a DIVA is about accepting and expecting the best of yourself.

3

DIVA: THE POWER SYSTEM

My friend Jim was pressing me one day. "What is it that you *really* want, Terri?" he asked. The answer flew out of my mouth without a thought: "I want to be a *diva*!"

We both laughed. The word *diva* conjured up such an overwhelming image of extravagant perfection, of extreme attitude: an opera singer like the late great Maria Callas, perhaps, or an incredible star like Barbra Streisand. Maybe I didn't have what it takes to be that kind of intense, larger-than-life presence. But later, as I thought more about it, I realized that the word *diva* was actually the perfect description for my aspiration.

Think about it. What is a diva? A diva is someone who is so *right* with herself and what she does that you can't imagine her in any other skin. She lives what she does. Aretha Franklin is a diva; can you imagine her doing anything besides singing? Peggy Fleming is a diva; she embodies the essence of figure skating. Barbara Walters is a diva; she inhabits her role of trusted television journalist with perfect ease. And that's what I wanted to strive for; I wanted to live with focus and attitude.

When I first introduced the concept of being a diva to my

students, none of them exactly did back flips to show their enthusiasm.

"What's the matter?" I asked. "Don't you want to be divas?"

"I don't," one woman answered. "Divas are snobs. You know, they're . . ."

"Bitches!" another woman exclaimed.

"They come in with too much attitude, like, 'I'm so hot,'" ventured another.

"So you hear the word *diva,* and it means a woman who has a superior attitude." I said. "She thinks she's the greatest. I wonder, what's so wrong with that? What if she can back it up? To me, a diva is a person who believes she's the best—who knows it, in fact, because she *is.* She always comes through. The thing is, if you're going to have the attitude, you'd better be able to deliver the goods.

"And let's talk about this rap of being a bitch. Why do you think women who accomplish awesome things are so often labeled bitches? Maybe it's because a person who excels is focused and intent on what she's doing. Some people are intimidated by that intensity of focus. If you lack it yourself, it's really hard to witness it and not feel either overpowered, jealous, or both. It's easy to point a finger and say, 'What a bitch!' That completely dismisses it, doesn't it? No one says Pavarotti or Placido Domingo is a bitch—or the male equivalent. But if a Kathleen Battle or Cecelia Bartoli behave the same way, everyone is after their heads."

You have to get past the put-downs and really see what is possible. Define *diva* for yourself. Being a diva is simply about being whole. It's knowing that your spirit, mind, and body are a complete, functional unit. In my fitness system, diva stands for *d*etermination, *i*ntegrity, *v*itality, and *a*spiration. The DIVA System begins with the understanding that every woman can become a champion. That means making the most of your life, body, and style. Learn to recognize and employ positive strategies that will help you to achieve your goals.

The champion's attitude is at the heart of DIVA. Physical strength and health are the keys to a sense of confidence that goes far beyond how you look. It's the underpinning to beauty. Start with how you feel. Do you feel strong, powerful, exuberant? I don't mean this in the sense that you can bench press your own weight but in the sense that you have a direction in life. Do you feel like your body is running clean—no drugs, alcohol, or chemicals? Do you feel comfortable in your own skin? Do you like the idea of exploring how you move through space? The DIVA System can help you develop the skills you need to accomplish that confidence.

Most women's fitness programs start with beauty. I start with strength. Strength is beautiful. Women dream of having extraordinary bodies that are lithe and tight and turn heads, and the fitness industry, cosmetics industry, and plastic surgeons all exist to cater to every aspect of that dream. But the truth is that there's only one real path to both beauty and fitness: It's getting strong.

It's not going to be fast or easy. This is no infomercial promise: "Great abs in two weeks . . . a shapely body in three minutes a day." The point is not to chase windmills. It's to integrate fitness into your life, to take joy in physical motion, to take pride in knowing your body can do what you need it to do.

The DIVA Path

At forty, Karen is lithe, strong, and fit. She exudes energy, confidence, youth, and joy. Being around her is an inspiration. But

Susan, who is thirty-two, had never worked out before because she always felt weak and clumsy. She described herself as a "fireplug." Now she says, "I realized right away that I wasn't weak and that it didn't matter if I looked stupid. No one was looking at me or judging me anyway. There were a lot of benefits that I didn't expect. I gained a new sense of self-confidence and pride. I saw that I could do anything if I worked hard enough at it."

....

Cara, who is twenty-nine, battled a weight problem all her life. Her goal had always been to get thin, and she was a chronic dieter. When she shift-ed her focus to getting strong, she found a new path. She says, "Dieting wasn't the issue anymore. Strength was. I really liked the feeling of empowerment, both physical and emotional. For the first time in my life, I felt proud to be in my body."

Karen would be the first to tell you that she didn't always have such a positive self-image. For most of her life, her pervasive feeling was one of vulnerability. She learned the message very young: *You aren't strong enough. You can't do it. You don't deserve it. Your goals are out of reach.*

In Karen's early twenties, her father died suddenly. Deeply dependent on him, she was traumatized to a state of near-helplessness. Her sense of failure was so ingrained in her that she felt personally responsible for his death. She was haunted by the thought that life was arbitrary and dangerous, and there was nothing she could do to control any of it. She became severely depressed.

A friend suggested that Karen take a dance class to cheer her up, and she reluctantly agreed. She certainly didn't expect much.

But the dance class did far more than cheer Karen up. She discovered that movement was a healing force for her. She learned that being in shape and in control of her body gave her the feeling that she could be in control of her life, too—that she didn't have to be swallowed alive by external events.

Karen explains it today in this way: "Through movement, I truly feel more integrated and more in touch with my strengths, and I have the motivation to master most situations I come across. My mental clarity, my thought processes, are much keener after I've moved."

Karen reminds me once again of the true power of fitness—how transformational and comprehensive strength and confidence can be for a woman. Yet the benefits of fitness are rarely cast in this light, as an inherent self-esteem booster. The self-esteem message is usually more along the lines of "Once you have a tight butt, everything else will be great." Oh, yeah. But you've got to have the tight butt first. I don't think that's much of a self-esteem message. Self-esteem should be unconditional: You're great because you're designed to be that way. It's natural.

Consider this new idea. You have probably found that most fitness programs are based on fixing what is wrong with you. They feed your insecurities: your fears of getting fat or looking flabby. My program is based on what's already right with you: your positives, not your negatives.

Here's the catch, though. If you want to be a Diva, you have to start with a different way of thinking. You're going to have to take a different attitude about your body, about the role of exercise, about what fitness means, and about who you are in your body. My method for training is born of an honest look at your own internal reality. By this I mean really examining yourself, thinking about the things you've never told anyone you're afraid of, and deciding to be strong.

I call it *reality thinking*. You must start living, thinking, breathing, being what you've set as your goal. You actually begin to metamorphosize into a Diva the moment you set it as your goal. Once you visualize a goal, you have started down the path of achieving that goal. The trick is to believe in yourself throughout the process.

Rachel, who is thirty-six, admitted that she had always felt intimidated by the fitness world. She wouldn't set foot into a gym because it seemed so competitive. After working with me for a few months, Rachel now says, "Women in this society have a choice about whether to buy into the fitness hype or not. We need to educate ourselves. There are so many intelligent options available to us now. I think it's a pretty weak excuse to just say you can't do it. It's no longer the dark ages in the world of exercise. I mean, it's up to you."

Skating Backward in the Dark

Several years ago I started Rollerblading. It was a new challenge, and I threw myself into it. Every day, I'd go over to Central Park and practice until I was confident enough to start skating on the streets of Manhattan. I'm always looking for ways to push myself, so once I was able to go forward pretty well, I started practicing skating backward.

It was hard: both disorienting and scary. I couldn't get a

sense of balance and flow because there were so many dangers. Then one night a couple of adventurous friends and I decided to go to the park and practice skating in the dark. I was amazed to find that I could skate backward a lot faster at night than I could during the day. At first I couldn't figure out why.

Then it hit me: When I could see all of the dangers, the roadblocks, the branches on the ground waiting to trip me up, I was unconsciously tightening up and hesitating, getting too involved in the danger of it. When I couldn't see the obstacles, I had to let go, loosen up, and just skate.

Working out and getting strong is a lot like that. Initially, your fears and negative self-perceptions are glittering in the light of day, and they seem to be part of everything you do. You approach the experience with some exaggerated picture in your head of how unbearable, painful, and humiliating it will be. I say: Hey, where did that come from? Some long-ago nightmare gym class? Maybe somebody said something to you once and you believed them. Maybe you had a bad experience—got tripped up. Whatever the source of this misconception, I'm here to tell you and to show you differently.

Denise, a new student of mine, had a very clear conception of herself. Her mother had always told her, "Denise, you're such a klutz." Believe me, Denise was loaded with self-doubt when she began working out. The first time she stumbled, she turned beet red and apologized, saying, "I'm sorry. I'm a real klutz."

"You are?" I asked. "How do you know that?"

Denise shrugged. "Well, look at the way I just tripped."

"Denise," I said, wanting to nip this klutz thing in the bud, "have you ever seen an Olympic ice skater fall on the ice?"

"Sure."

"Do you say, 'Boy, what a klutz!'"

Denise laughed. "Oh, no. They've practiced for years. They slip . . ." Denise paused and smiled at me. She was starting to get my point.

"When you're training, you make mistakes, you fall down, you trip. It's part of the process. It's the same thing a baby does when she's learning to walk."

I encouraged Denise to forget about labeling herself, to stop expecting immediate perfection, to forget about being Denise the Klutz. Now she could focus on the work instead of the negative picture she always kept in her head.

It's just too easy to let other people define you. But your confidence, your strength, and your physical power belong to you.

Meet the DIVAs

Every day, I see the evidence of success in the women who work with me and have chosen to explore the DIVA path. Their testimonials to the power of the DIVA System confirm my belief that we are entering a new era of fitness for women.

These are ordinary women, not the hard-core fitness junkies that fill the gyms and scare people away from exploring their own strengths. They are women who never before dared to see themselves as strong. They were afraid of their power. Now, they luxuriate in it. They have come to believe that power is totally feminine and beautiful.

Being a DIVA is about living your life and developing confidence in your physicality. Squats, push-ups, and abdominal crunches aren't unrelated exercises. You'll learn that every movement you make in the course of a day is based on a squat (sitting down in a chair or jumping over a puddle), a push-up (lifting a box onto a shelf), and an abdominal crunch (picking up a baby). It is shocking to me that many women actually feel shaky on their feet: ungrounded, unsteady, and afraid of movement.

With the DIVA System, your body will soon begin to feel strong. Believe me, it's a great feeling!

4
EVERYBODY STARTS AS A BEGINNER

We're such a nation of experts! Everyone walks around thinking she should know it all. It's embarrassing to admit that you're a beginner. You think, "I'm an adult. I should know."

The first step in the DIVA process is to find out what you don't know. Accept the interesting idea that you're a beginner. It will free you from needing to be an expert. You may be feeling nervous about the unknown, but rest assured that it's great to start from the beginning. It's great to realize that you're not expected to know, produce, or win. As a beginner, you have the freedom to explore how your body works, with no preconceived notions of the outcome. You're just learning, and you'll discover a surprising strength and energy in that state.

This may be an entirely new idea for you. Why? Because everyone around you is always trying to push you to know and produce and win. It takes a real inner power to say, "Get off my back and let me learn this!"

The wonderful secret of being a beginner is that there is no such thing as *trying* to do something. The very instant you start, you're already *doing* it. Even if you get stuck or frustrated, you're still *doing* it. The only remaining issue is your *skill* level, which keeps getting better the more you practice.

As you keep repeating each exercise, building the skill, it will become ingrained in your motor memory, the same way that ideas become ingrained in your consciousness. Accepting the beginner status and finding out what you don't know will free your mind to accept the changes you have set for yourself.

Maybe it's hard to think you deserve to treat yourself well. When you say, "I don't have time to exercise," maybe what you're really saying is, "I'm not good enough to make time for myself."

The DIVΛ System is self-exploration through physical means. Personalize your goal and think of how to access it. Resist looking outside yourself for answers.

Find Your True Motivation

Sometimes our motivation for change may stem from a desire not to face some reality about ourselves. Maybe subconsciously you're thinking, "I can't control my relationship or job. At least I'll be able to control my body."

It's not my place to tell you that there is a right motivation and a wrong motivation or to preach about how you should feel. But it's important for you to know where your motivation is coming from. For example, when I started out, my motivation was that I wanted to *look* strong. When I really thought about it, it came down to the decidedly unglamorous reason of being afraid. I was afraid all the time. I was afraid that if my stepfather was in a good mood, he'd want to "be nice." I was afraid that if he was in a bad mood, he'd beat me.

I kept thinking that if I looked strong, maybe he (and later, other evil-minded people who might come into my life) would leave me alone. My desire to be strong was not born of some far-flung idea. It came from a basic survival instinct.

My survival instinct grew into a burning desire to change the way I dealt with the world and the way the world dealt with me. I was able to turn my motivation of fear into positive action. I wasn't always consciously aware of this, but as I grew stronger, I developed understanding. My motivation became clear.

The point is, don't try to hide your motivation for change. Just acknowledge the real reason, no matter how unsavory or even vain it may be. Then, as you start to train, reassess your motivation as you go. You'll find that sometimes you'll experience positive feelings about yourself, and sometimes you'll experience negative feelings about yourself. And once you really see that you're worth it, and know that you'll keep going, that initial motivation will become the turning point that you'll refer to later on.

Lee, a student of many years, is an example of this transformation. Her decision to work out came from a humiliating moment. One morning while she was standing nude in the bathroom brushing her hair, her husband came up behind her and exclaimed with alarm, "Lee, your ass fell!" Lee was devastated. Suddenly she felt ugly and unworthy. The next day, she showed up at my door ready to work out.

When I remind Lee today of her initial motivation, she just laughs. She is no longer the woman whose confidence can be shaken with a rude remark. She has discovered another dimension to her world: a strength that makes her less vulnerable to humiliation. Many of my students report the same experience.

"I went away to college and my friends started dating and I got tired of myself and my negative notions about myself. I decided it was time for a change. I was hiding behind an exterior where I didn't have to let people in until I was 'perfect' but I knew, always, that I was already special and talented, but not many other people knew that because I didn't project it. So my motivation was to be accepted. Now I see it a different way. By working out, I learned to feel and to project my power."

Patty, 25

"When I was twenty-eight, someone told me that everyone's metabolism slows down at thirty. Since I loved to eat, and was thin, I didn't want to have to change my eating habits at thirty, so I began to work out to attempt to keep my metabolism going. Now, seven years later, my motivation is to feel good. Looking good is nice, but what I really love, and what keeps me going back to the gym day after day is how I feel after a workout. I feel strong, happy, and confident. Like I could do anything!"

Lois, 35

Begin to Feel Your Power

Every woman, regardless of her age, athletic ability, and history, can recover the power that is her birthright. Looking good is a wonderful side effect of the real benefit: being a stronger, happier, you.

Before you start the DIVA System, take a few minutes for an honest look at yourself, your fears, and your goals. Chances are, the very things that have been standing in the way of achieving fitness goals are the same barriers that prevent success in your career, relationships, and other areas of your life. My goal is to shatter all of those barriers. In a sense, your fitness goals become a metaphor for your life. So, take a few moments to reflect on these questions and answer them for yourself. (You might want to save your answers and look at them again in six months. I'll bet you won't recognize yourself!)

YOUR PERSONAL SURVEY

1. Describe the negative impressions you've always had about your body. For example, "I'm too fat." "My legs are stubby." "I'm weak." Do you hate something about the way you look? Do you wish you had someone else's body?

2. Do you dread exercising or feel that it's something you can't really do well? If so, where did those impressions come from? Describe your experience. Maybe you were told you couldn't do something. Or you tried and failed, so you were always reluctant to try again.

3. What is your motivation for fitness? (Be honest! Don't avoid facing it, even if it sounds silly.)

4. Describe your expectations of this training.

5. Describe your fears going in. For example, are you afraid you won't last, that you'll quit, that there will be too much pain, that you'll look foolish, that you'll fail?

6. What do you think it would take to feel good about yourself—to feel like a success?

While you are working on the DIVA System, keep your survey in the forefront and watch for the changes that are occurring within and without. Throughout the book, I'll offer dozens of tips to keep you motivated and positively oriented. And I'll share the experiences many of my clients have had in their quest to become DIVAs.

Before You Begin

Take a look at what you'll need to guarantee success. This is a big journey, and you never take a big journey without being well prepared. Here are the basics.

A PHYSICAL CHECKUP

Never start an exercise regimen without knowing your real physical shape. That doesn't mean how you look; it means what your physical condition is. Do this first, whether you're twenty-five or fifty, thin or overweight, generally healthy or prone to illness. It's the safe, sensible, and sane way to make sure you can do this without any problems. It's also a great way to get the information you need as a starting point for your new regimen.

A MOTIVATIONAL ENVIRONMENT

I want you to think about the space you're going to use for the DIVA work. Consider this with as much care as you would use when choosing a place to live. This space, large or small, is going to be the home for your new self.

If you have a room in your house or apartment that you can devote to your work, that's great. But it works just as well if you only have the corner of a room. Lay down a carpet or use heavy tape to define the area you'll be using. Try to give yourself an 8' × 10' area. If that's not possible, aim for a 6' × 9' area. Remember, you're not going to be standing still. Try to also find a place to keep your supplies: a towel, a floor mat, and the equipment I'll suggest.

If you can, only use this space for your workouts. Add features that are motivational for you: music, a certain kind of light, a picture on the wall. The important thing is to create a space that draws you into it—a place that you love to go.

A REALISTIC SCHEDULE

If you've ever tried and failed to stick with an exercise plan, I'll bet one of the factors was schedule. You promised yourself you'd work for a certain amount of time first thing in the morning or after work or whenever. But life kept getting in the way.

Be honest and realistic from the start. Don't set yourself up for failure. Decide.

- What time of day feels best for exercising?
- What time of day is most convenient for your schedule?
- Are there certain days of the week that are crowded with activities that would make it harder to exercise?

10.00
chapters
1998

613.7045
Wal

518517

- In the beginning (say, the first month), how many days a week are you going to commit to? Three? Four?
- What time frame are you going to set aside? A half hour? Forty-five minutes?

Once you figure out the best schedule, write it down. Be sure to make it flexible—such as, two to four times a week instead of just four.

THE RIGHT DRESS

Choose roomy, comfortable clothes and strong, flexible sneakers. Clothes should allow a full range of motion and not inhibit any part of your body. Wear a sports bra or a bra with good support. Pull your hair out of your face. Keep a towel and water bottle handy.

The most important clothing item is your shoes. Wear cross-training or basketball shoes, not running shoes. Running shoes have a waffle pattern that's easy to trip on if you wear them for workouts. The best aerobic or walking shoe has cushioning, stabilizing features at the ankles, and flexibility in the toes and heels. Try on various brands until you find the perfect fit—not too tight and not too loose. Never do a workout in bare feet, socks, or street shoes.

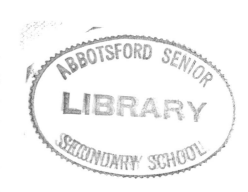

BASIC EQUIPMENT

This is important. Your commitment to the DIVA System requires that you get some basic equipment. It's not expensive or complicated, but these items will be necessary to attain full mastery of the exercises. Here's what you'll need:

1. Two sets of dumbbells, five pounds and ten pounds

You can get dumbbells (also called free weights) at a department store or a sporting goods store. Try different styles to find the ones that feel most comfortable in your hands. If you have never worked with dumbbells before, you might want to start with two pounds instead of five pounds.

2. A power band

This is a big, fat rubber band to be used for stretching and balancing exercises. It can also provide resistance in other exercises. Power bands are available inexpensively at most sporting goods stores. Since there are different styles and thicknesses, check them out before you choose. Find one that seems durable and doesn't hurt your hand when you grasp it firmly. (Once you purchase a band, treat it with care and it will last longer. Avoid snagging it on rings or fingernails, and keep it in a cool, dry place.)

3. A six- to eight-foot exercise bar

Sure, you can use a heavy mop handle, if you want. But an actual exercise bar is preferable, and again, not expensive. Be sure it's not too heavy, because the point in the beginning will be balance and form, not strength. However, you may wish to invest a few extra dollars to get a bar that comes with removable weight plates so you can add weight as you advance. (If necessary, the dumbbells can be used instead of a bar.)

4. A sturdy low bench or stool

Be sure it's sturdy enough to climb onto without tipping it over. A commercial aerobic step unit is a good alternative. In the beginning, you can also use the bottom step of a staircase.

5. A full-length mirror

Until you learn to feel when your body is in the correct position, a mirror will help you see it and make quick corrections.

A Word About Machines

Sometimes I'm asked, "What's the point of working so hard when you can just go to a gym and use any of dozens of machines?" I use machines very, very little—hardly at all, if I can help it. Machines may seem to help you work more effectively, but what they really do is take over the work that your smaller stabilizing muscles have to do. Your major muscle groups get stronger and stronger, but the smaller muscle groups don't get used.

For example, your abdominals can become very weak by working on machines. Most people don't innately know to pull them in when they do the motion. There was a time I used to do a lot of machine work, and I got very strong. But guess what? When I tried to stand on one leg and balance myself, I couldn't do it. You can use those inner thigh machines until you turn blue, but it won't help your balance.

Also, if you want to do any movement that requires forward motion—like Rollerblading or ice skating—you need to be able to transfer your weight onto one leg and stay there for a minute. Even riding a bike requires balance at the center of your body.

The whole torso is your power center. You won't learn how that feels from a machine.

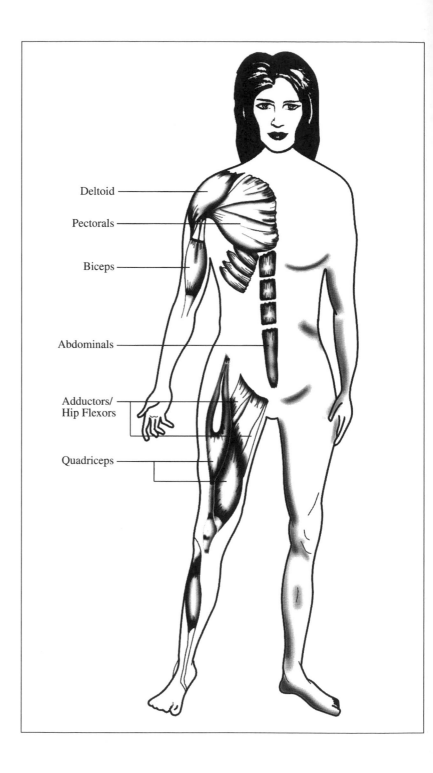

Deltoid

Pectorals

Biceps

Abdominals

Adductors/
Hip Flexors

Quadriceps

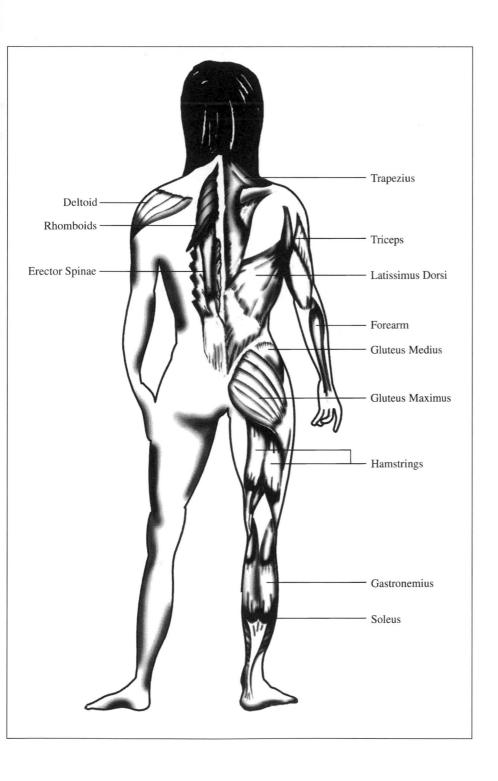

Deltoid

Rhomboids

Erector Spinae

Trapezius

Triceps

Latissimus Dorsi

Forearm

Gluteus Medius

Gluteus Maximus

Hamstrings

Gastronemius

Soleus

Make a Contract with Yourself

What does it take to make the commitment? It takes only your decision to do it. Writing it down will make it more tangible. In your journal, write these words, then sign and date it:

> I am willing to truly be who I am.
> To use *myself* as my own true ideal.
> To give myself the benefit of the doubt.
> To let myself struggle without giving up.
> To keep going, with small, consistent steps.
> To remind myself that life is happening *now,* not in the future.

PART 2

THE
DIVA
WORK

5
STRENGTH, BALANCE, ENERGY . . . LIFE!

Many women get discouraged when they exercise because they never learned to use their bodies. From early on, they heard the message, "You can't do that," or "Girls shouldn't do that," or "That's not ladylike." That message took root and remained at the core of their self-image.

Sharon, a forty-year-old student, told me how it happened for her. "When I was growing up, there were two kinds of girls: those who used their bodies and those who used their minds," Sharon recalled. The former group played volleyball, hiked, and ice skated. The latter went to the library and the theater.

"I was in the latter group. I didn't use my body because, frankly, I didn't want to be considered stupid—a girl jock. No one ever told me, and it never occurred to me on my own, that my body was more than an appendage to my brain. I didn't relate being able to do things with my body to real life. It might have really started at puberty, when my mother told me matter-of-factly, 'You can't run or climb trees anymore. You're a woman now.' After that, I always thought only the dumb or mannish women were active. I thought I had to make a choice between being smart and womanly or being active and manly. It's a shame I never learned the truth—that the integration of mind and body is what makes for strength, health, longevity, and intelligence."

Sharon regretted the lost years when she might have been achieving a certain strength and surety in her body. But still, even at age forty, she plunged in. She spoke honestly about how she overcame her fears.

"The women in my family have always been short and broad-hipped," Sharon said. "Lush-looking in youth, they all succumbed to an inevitable spread as they aged. I expected to follow this pattern, too. I was resigned to being plump and matronly by the time I reached my fifties. As I began to exercise, I had to come to terms with my self-doubt and feelings of inadequacy about using my body. I really wondered if it was possible for me to get fit at this point, to do these exercises without killing myself from the exertion, and to see any visible results. My biggest fear was that it was too late for me."

Sharon stuck with it. I'm proud of the way she has evolved into a fully physical being. Her words got me to thinking that her attitudes about being physical were not that uncommon for women. Movement is as natural as life itself, yet all these women are walking around saying to themselves, "I'm not a physical person."

What Sharon learned—and you will learn, too—is that exercise is not just physical. You're thinking all the time. Thinking intensely. Exercise is simply knowledge in action. As you work, your mind and body will actively begin to merge. You will easily and naturally start putting what you're learning into practice. Take it slow and allow yourself to acclimate to the changes. We're going to go through each exercise step-by-step, fully learning and understanding the movements before we put them into a program. You'll notice that as your understanding increases, so will your strength. As your intensity and competence increase, you'll begin to feel the effects in other areas of your life.

Keep in mind as you go that experiencing determination, integrity, vitality, and aspiration in your life is what this system is all about. Exercise is not just something you do in the gym or at home. It's utterly vital to life—as essential as learning to walk, run, or jump.

Don't allow your initial confusion about your goals or a fear of failure to paralyze you. Stop looking ahead to the moment you might fail, and keep your attention focused in the now—each moment of discovery. Think of your big goal as an umbrella, and each small step as a spoke in that umbrella. Confront each challenge as you face it. Don't worry about the results. They will happen. Trust the method. Trust yourself. This is what's required in order to proceed:

1. You'll need an understanding of how your body works as a total unit. Stop seeing yourself as a collection of body parts and think instead of your body as a functional, vibrant unit.
2. A basic knowledge of alignment and correct form is also essential. Form and technique are the keys to success. Your body develops the way you carry it.
3. Finally, you must have a general understanding of why things are done the way they are.

That's the learning process.

The DIVA Workout

The DIVA body is the practical and visible manifestation of the DIVA System. The workouts in this section are your route to becoming a DIVA in action.

This is a simple program that includes four clearly defined sections, each containing four targeted exercises. You can better grasp the role of each exercise by knowing which section it belongs in: Determination, Integrity, Vitality, or Aspiration.

DETERMINATION: to build strength

INTEGRITY: to achieve stability and balance

VITALITY: to create energy and agility

ASPIRATION: to develop flexibility and cardiovascular fitness

The format of the Determination, Integrity, Vitality, and Aspiration workouts is a simple, easy-to-follow method that includes a practical, usable technique as well as a motivational (or emotional) underpinning. It's important that you know what you're doing, why you're doing it, and what you can hope to achieve. It's all outlined here. With only sixteen basic exercises, you can achieve all of your goals.

I've designed this system to make it easy for you to do on your own. I know it's sometimes hard when you're looking at a tape or reading a book to follow exactly what you should be doing—how your body is positioned, what the move looks like. That's why I've broken each exercise down into many simple steps.

This section explains how to do each exercise and answers basic questions that often arise. The next section lays it all out in workouts and an eating plan suitable for a one-year goal.

There are four stages to the system. I call them progressions because each one represents a progression to a new level.

- Progression One teaches you the basics of doing each exercise.
- Progression Two begins to incorporate the exercises into workouts and introduces the nutritional component.
- Progression Three offers advanced and more challenging combinations and requires more strength and speed.
- Progression Four gives you the opportunity to take what you've learned and create your own exercise pattern, including picking a sport or activity that will get you out into the world.

Before you start, sit down and read through the entire book to get an idea of what to expect: What's involved in each exercise? How do I begin? What's the point of each progression? How do I use the journal? And so on.

I know you're probably thinking, Why a *year*? Why not six weeks or three months or something you can jump in and out of for quick results. First, I don't believe in doing anything halfway—especially when it comes to being a DIVA. Second, you will see results right away.

Every single time you do a workout, something will be different. Movements that were nearly impossible the first time will seem a bit easier the second time, and easier still the third time. You'll increase the weight you lift. You'll be faster and do more repetitions.

If you're consistent—let me say it again—*if you're consistent,* you'll see the biggest changes in the first three months. I realize that sometimes it's not so easy to be consistent. Even consistency is a skill you'll have to learn. So, I've designed the system to run over the space of one year so you can find your own pace. There's no one-size-fits-all time frame for everyone. *You* decide the time and pace at which to set your goals. *You* decide when you're ready to increase your intensity. *You* decide when you're ready to move on to the next level.

You own this system. You inhabit it. It's yours. There's no judge or jury or fitness maniac telling you that you've fallen behind on the course. There's only one way: *your* way. There's only one pace: *your* pace. There's only one person to please: *you.*

You might wonder what happens if you're inconsistent. Absolutely everyone is inconsistent sometimes. We're just humans, after all. But you will find that over time, as you begin to see results, you will feel differently, and your need to treat yourself well will outweigh your need to slow yourself down. It will come naturally.

Once you achieve understanding with one step, there will be a gradual, natural progression to the next step. You'll know when you're ready to move on, because you'll naturally ask the questions that get you to the next level. Your body will tell you that you're ready. This is the beginning of confidence. When you listen to your own body and mind and trust the message you're receiving, you begin to own your physical life. While your confidence builds through exercise, you'll find it automatically appearing in other areas of your life.

- You'll become more confident at work.
- You'll leave relationships where you are not treated with respect.
- You'll stop envying the way other women look; it will be fine to be just you.

- You'll develop an inner sense that all is right with the world—and with you.
- You'll no longer feel so afraid to try something new.

So, let's get started!

6

DETERMINATION

Consider the women you know or have seen in movies or read about in books who have determination. What do you notice about them? What sets them apart? Probably the first thing you'd say is, "They're strong women." And you may really admire that quality, but you may have no idea how to achieve it yourself.

> **Write down your female role models for Determination. Who are the strong ones?**

Determination is the key to strength. It's the will to change and the commitment to keep working in spite of setbacks. As you perform the Determination workout, you may find some fears surfacing that you didn't know you had: the fear of pain, the fear of experiencing your own power, the fear of strength.

Strength is not a dirty word for women. It doesn't mean bulging muscles or hair on your face or a manly gait. The secret to a healthy, graceful body is a strong and balanced center. All

> *"Determination is looking and feeling strong. I like the fact that I'm more self-sufficient: I can lift heavier things, move furniture, run without getting breathless. I don't like being helpless or dependent."*
>
> *Coleen, 24*

....

> *"I didn't used to feel very good about myself. Working out gave me confidence in my ability to achieve things I thought were impossible. It has also helped me to accept myself just as I am. Everyone has good character traits and less desirable character traits, good physical features and less attractive features. I've seen how important it is to accept both sides of yourself. Women tend to focus on their less attractive qualities and to overlook their good points. This seems self-defeating—and sad."*
>
> *Tara, 32*

improvements begin with strength. If you want smaller thighs, get stronger. If you want a trimmer waistline, get stronger. If you want a tighter butt or better posture, get stronger. There is absolutely no goal that cannot be reached by becoming stronger.

The result of strength is confidence, which means that you believe in your success. This may seem obvious, but I'm always amazed that women's negative perceptions of their bodies become such a part of them that they can't even see positive change when it happens. Recently, a student of mine was complaining because after several months of hard work, she didn't think her body looked any different. I took a tape measure and checked it out. She had lost five inches in her butt, yet she couldn't see it. She was so used to failure that she was blind to success. Needless to say, she was amazed when she saw the truth on the tape measure.

The goal of strength-building exercises is to build your physical presence in the world and your mental strength so that it lives in your body. Have you ever seen a woman walk into a room and been impressed with the strength of her presence? Maybe she wasn't beautiful in any standard way, but there was something powerful about her. That's the goal of strength-building exercises.

Determination exercises do more than just strengthen your body. They force you to strengthen your mind. It has to happen together, or none of it will. Your results correlate directly with how far you are willing to take your mind and your belief in yourself. There is absolutely nothing you can't do if you really want to.

Women often have a hard time accepting their achievements, acknowledging that they've done well, and giving themselves credit. What happened to the idea of standing up and getting your award when you win? It's a lost concept for many women, and that's why I teach confidence along with strength.

The exercises that represent Determination:

1. Push-up
2. Shoulder press
3. Stiff-legged deadlift
4. Lunge

"There's a certain transference of power from becoming stronger physically to both work and social contact. When I accomplish something new physically, it's like 'I can do that' and maybe there are other things that I can do. For example: 'I'm not going to work for a lower rate, because I'm worth my full rate.' 'This person is not going to put me down because I'm strong, I'm good, I'm great!' Also, if I'm ever feeling down or badly about the way something went, a good workout is my antidote. It makes me feel positive and also gives me that 'mind-clearing' . . . if only for an hour or so. The mind-clearing time has been a lifesaver for me."
Michelle, 34

"When faced with adversity, it is better to take a dance class, exercise, or get out on the tennis court than to pop a Valium. We need to learn constructive ways to feel our strength and power and hold onto ourselves."
Grace, 39

PUSH-UP

My female students often tell me that they consider push-ups a man's exercise. A lot of them have never even attempted to do a push-up. When I ask why, they respond that men are more capable of performing such a muscular exercise without even really trying.

"Hey, since when are push-ups gender-specific?" I ask. "If you think those muscles are weak, what better reason to develop them?"

Push-ups are the first exercise I teach women because of the gym class syndrome of not being able to do hard exercises. I want to eliminate that barrier right away. When you do a push-up, even if it's hard for you, you almost instantly get a glimpse of the power that is lying dormant within you. It's an exhilarating experience to do something you never thought you could do. In most cases, I get at least one push-up from a student in her first or second class.

Before you can attempt a straight-leg push-up, make sure you can do a basic version that will give you a lot more control of the whole process. The only change will be that your knees will be bent and resting on the floor instead of straight out behind you.

Muscles Involved

Major: chest (pectorals), deltoid, triceps
Stabilizing: shoulders, back, lower body, abdomen

These are the muscles that are used. Looks like a lot, doesn't it? Push-ups are usually thought of as just for your upper body, but you're actually using your whole body. I teach push-ups as a full-body exercise because many muscles are acting in sync to perform the motion. You can't do a push-up one muscle at a time.

Benefits (Why You Do a Push-Up)

➤ Prevents a jiggly upper arm. Remember, your tricep is the upper two-thirds of the back of your arm. If the muscles are strong, your arm won't sag.

➤ Strengthens your triceps, shoulders, and chest. Practically, that means any time you need to lift something over your head or push something away from you, you'll have the strength to do it.

➤ Teaches the idea of the integration of all your muscles.

➤ Involves the utilization of your abdominals and lower body as stabilizers. That means you work those areas without isolating them, just by tightening them.

You Will Need

➤ A floor mat or towel

WHAT IS THE RIB CAGE HINGE?

When you're in a normal position—just walking down the street or sitting in a chair, your rib cage is *open*. The motion of pulling your abdominal muscles and your navel in and back closes the hinge that keeps your rib cage open. Imagine pulling your navel straight in toward the back of your body.

How to Do the Exercise

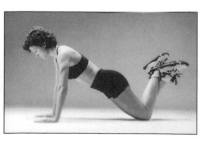
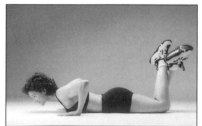
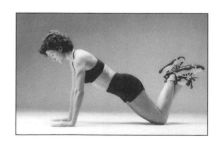

Position

1. Lie flat on the floor, facedown.
2. Cross your ankles and bend your knees.
3. Relax your shoulders down.
4. Stretch your neck long.
5. Place your hands shoulder width apart and spread your fingers.
6. Squeeze your legs together, and tighten your butt.
7. Pull your abs and navel in—close the rib cage hinge.

Motion

1. Take a deep breath. As if you're gripping the floor with your hands, *push* the floor away, keeping your body flat and straight like a tabletop. Exhale as you push. Then lower yourself to the floor and repeat. Exhale when pushing. Inhale when lowering.
2. Go all the way down and touch the floor between each repetition. You can lie down if you need to and start each repetition fresh. The most important thing is to get a full range of motion—meaning the full extent of the motion throughout a joint. In this case, the full length of your arms.
3. Practice the motion a few times, checking your form, until you feel comfortable with the exercise. Relax, take a break, then try it again. Your goal is three sets of ten repetitions.

   ADVANCED: Same as above, but straighten your legs and squeeze them together. Again, go all the way to the floor if you need to, but touch the floor with the entire front of your body.

DIVA Secrets

✓ Think of a push-up as *pushing* the floor away, not pulling your body up.

✓ Make your hands an active part of the move. They're not just lying there on the floor. They're *gripping* the floor to push it away.

✓ Avoid having a turtle neck. Keep your neck long and shoulders down. If your shoulders are up by your jawline, they're too high.

✓ When you're doing a push-up correctly, your body feels like a board—all in one piece. You have a sense of connection, a muscular tension that keeps you from being loose and floppy.

DIVA Troubleshooter

• I feel pain in my hands and a strain in my wrists when I do a push-up. What's wrong?

First, check the position of your hands to be sure they are located under your shoulders. If they're too far forward, you'll feel a strain in your wrists. Also, check to make sure you're not riding your hands (letting all of your weight push into your hands) instead of using them to grip and push away the floor.

• How do I know I'm engaging my abs properly?

You know your abs are connected when the rib cage hinge is closed. (see sidebar on page fifty-five.) It is also part of the connection you will feel when you're performing the exercise correctly. Your abs will want to be in place while they're working. Your body will feel like a single piece, with no sag in the middle.

A WORD ABOUT BREATHING

Some beginners automatically hold their breath when they're exerting themselves, which is exactly the opposite of what they should be doing. When you breathe, you send oxygen to your muscles, enabling them to do the work. I'm not talking about little, ladylike breaths. I'm talking about big whooshing inhalations and exhalations. It should feel like a routine: *Inhale . . . exhale as you push . . . inhale . . . exhale as you push.* If you start to feel dizzy while doing an exercise, chances are you're not breathing.

....

"We acquire the strength we have overcome."

Ralph Waldo Emerson

• **I have a hard time lifting my body because my arms feel too weak.**

Some women just don't have any muscularity in their upper bodies when they begin. In time, with practice, you'll gradually begin to develop muscles. However, it helps to keep the focus off your arms. You aren't lifting your body with your arms, you're pushing the floor away. Also check to make sure you're squeezing your legs together. If you are, you won't experience a disjointed or awkward lifting sensation. Your body will feel like one piece.

• **What do you mean by a "full range of motion"?**

In a push-up, a full range of motion is equal to the entire length of your arms, from the floor to straight (not locked) elbows.

SHOULDER PRESS

The shoulder press builds stability as well as strength in your upper body. Why is that important? Once again, think of the way you present yourself when you're walking down the street. Do you look strong and confident, or do you look as if a faint breeze would knock you over? This is a helpful image to carry with you. Notice how you're moving the next time you're walking down the street. Which style do you present to the world?

My students have remarked that doing shoulder presses offers a deep internal sense of "I can *shoulder* my burdens. I can *push* the bad stuff away. I can *lift* my arms to the sky." When we're performing this exercise in a group, we always play uplifting music in sync with the motion. It's exhilarating! This sense of strength is very significant for women. The shoulder press represents overcoming the frailty in your upper body as well as the frailty in your mind.

Muscles Involved

Major: deltoids (front, rear, lateral), rhomboids, trapezius, triceps
Stabilizing: chest, back, abs, legs, feet, toes (if standing)

The shoulder press stabilizes your chest and back as it works your upper-body muscles in a balanced manner.

Benefits (Why You Do a Shoulder Press)

➤ Teaches the natural ease of posture balance.
➤ Projects a more stable, powerful person.

➤ Gives you aesthetically well-developed shoulders.

➤ Makes your waist and hips look smaller.

➤ Gives the appearance of straighter, longer arms and back.

➤ Enables you to be more graceful.

You Will Need

➤ Two dumbbells (start with two or five pounds)

➤ A low bench or chair

Position

1. Sit upright on a bench or a chair that is low enough for your feet to comfortably rest on the floor.

2. Plant your feet firmly on the floor, legs together.

How to Do the Exercise

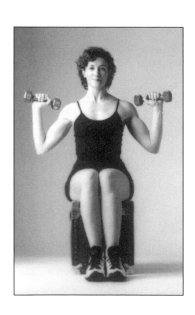
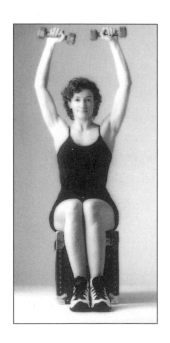
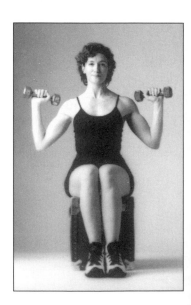

3. Hold a dumbbell in each hand with your palms facing outward.

4. Press your elbows against the sides of your body.

5. Lengthen your upper body by pulling in your abs and navel, relaxing your shoulders, and elongating your neck (as though someone was pulling your head straight toward the ceiling with a string).

Motion

1. Take a deep breath; on the exhale, push the weights up until your arms are almost straight (but not locked).

2. As you inhale, pull your arms down until your knuckles are almost level with the tops of your shoulders.

3. Repeat several times at a moderate pace. Keep checking your form—and don't forget to breathe. When you're comfortable with the form and motion, begin to increase the number of sets and gradually add weight. Your goal is three sets of ten repetitions.

VARIATION (STANDING): It is harder for many people to perform a standing shoulder press because it requires a strict lower-body position—meaning more energy and balance. However, not everyone responds to exercise in exactly the same way. Some people find the standing shoulder press easier because they can use their legs and torso to help stabilize and push the dumbbells upward.

STANDING SHOULDER PRESS
1. Stand straight, with your hips in line with your shoulders.
2. Plant your hips under your shoulders and pull in your navel.

3. Place your feet hip width apart, knees slightly bent, with knees and toes facing forward.

4. Perform the shoulder press as described above.

DIVA Secrets

✓ Concentrate on maintaining a straight alignment. The trick is keeping your neck long and your eyes forward, as though your head is gently being pulled upward by a string attached to the crown of your head. (If you want to know what that looks like, imagine a ballerina dancing *Swan Lake*.)

✓ Hold the dumbbells firmly, with your elbows tucked so your hands and arms don't wobble and throw you off balance. If your arm is pitching out sideways, you're not using correct alignment.

✓ Be as attentive to the form and motion coming down as you are pushing up. Don't flop the weights down; rather, the motion should feel like you are *pulling down*.

✓ Be careful not to jerk. Control the weight on the way up and on the way down.

✓ Although the movement is straight up, it's normal to feel as if your arms are going very slightly forward.

✓ When you're doing a standing shoulder press, check to make sure your hips are facing straight forward. It's not always easy to feel it in the beginning, so look in a mirror.

✓ If your legs are too far apart, your lower back may sag. They should be hip width apart.

DIVA Troubleshooter

"Energy . . . will remove mountains."
Hosea Balou

• I feel a strain in my elbows and back.

Check your position. Are you locking your elbows when you press the weights upward? Elbows should be very slightly bent. Also make sure that you're sitting or standing properly and your lower back isn't arched. An arched back can create an imbalance, putting pressure on and stressing muscles that are meant to be used as stabilizers. (Check the mirror if you're not sure.) An arched back may also mean that your abdominals are not engaged correctly.

• My upper body feels wobbly, like I'm going to tip over.

Is your rib cage hinge closed? (That is, your abdominal muscles are pulled in and your navel is pulled back toward your spine.) Make sure your hipbones are straight and level. Make sure you haven't added weight until your form is perfect. Make sure your feet are properly positioned. If you're standing, your knees should be slightly bent, with legs and knees in line with your hips. If you're seated, make sure your weight is perfectly distributed on the bench and that both feet are planted firmly on the floor.

• I feel OK when I'm pushing the weights *up*, but on the way down, I don't feel as much control.

That's because you think the real work is pushing up, and you automatically begin to let up when the weights are coming down. The control should be consistent both ways. It might help to imagine the movement as *pushing* up and *pulling* down.

GOOD PAIN/BAD PAIN

How do you know the difference between good pain (which means your muscles are working) and bad pain (which means you're hurting yourself)? The primary muscle groups being exercised will respond by feeling hot, sore and by slowing down as they grow tired. This is normal discomfort. If a muscle or a group of muscles causes you sharp, localized pain, stop immediately. You have pulled, stretched, or twisted where you shouldn't have. If the pain continues for an extended period, see a doctor.

• How do I know I'm ready to move on to a standing shoulder press?

Your body will tell you. Once you've mastered the form and are holding your body correctly, you won't feel the strain and sense of imbalance you feel when you're beginning. Form is the absolute key. When your form is off, everything feels harder than it actually is. The exercise isn't strengthening; it is ultimately self-defeating.

STIFF-LEGGED DEAD LIFT

I like to think of this as an active stretch. In other words, your entire body is working in an integrated way.

This exercise works the hamstrings and the entire back. You may feel a stretching sensation in your hamstrings and through the length of your back. This may be a little uncomfortable if you're not used to working these parts of your body, but it shouldn't be painful. Discomfort is a natural feeling when you're working your muscles. In time, you will become in tune with your body and know the difference between healthy discomfort and dangerous pain.

Muscles Involved

Hamstrings, back (upper and lower), triceps, deltoids

Benefits (Why You Do a Dead Lift)

➤ Prevents and/or corrects muscle imbalances—such as lower back pain—caused by weakness.
➤ Helps you develop total body coordination.
➤ Provides an excellent stretch for your hamstrings.

You Will Need

➤ A weighted exercise bar

Position

1. Stand straight, with your legs straight, positioned together or slightly apart, and your feet planted firmly on the floor. Your knees should be straight but not locked.
2. Hold a bar in both hands, knuckles facing outward, elbows straight, in front of your body at waist level. The bar should touch the tops of your thighs.
3. Pull abs in and back.
4. Elongate your neck and relax your shoulders. (In other words, don't hunch. Feel energy traveling up from the ground through your body.

Motion

1. Keeping your head up, bend slowly at the hip joint. (Think of sticking out your butt.) If you're bending from the waist, you're doing it wrong.

How to Do the Exercise

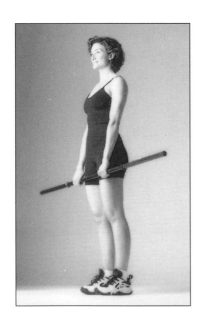
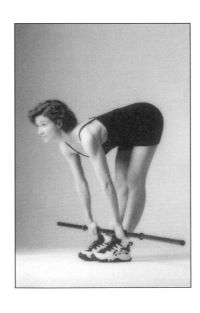
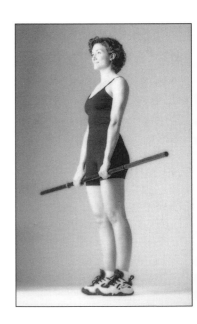

2. Try to touch the bar to the top of your ankles, keeping your back flat. You may not be able to go all the way down to your ankles and still keep your back flat. That's okay. Go as far as you can.

3. Keep your eyes looking straight ahead as you quickly stand up straight, maintaining a flat upper body. Think of your hamstrings pulling up into your butt.

4. Do not pull your arms up. Keep them close to the front of your body, with the stabilizing tension of your shoulders pressing back and down. (This is called engaging your upper back.)

5. Repeat the motion ten times. Your goal is three sets of ten repetitions.

DIVA Secrets

✓ When you're standing back up, imagine that your hamstrings are shades that you're pulling up into your butt. This action will keep your body flat, not hunched.

✓ Push your feet into the floor to engage your muscles and start the movement.

✓ Your back should look like the flat top of a table, not rounded.

✓ Be sure to bend from the hip joint, not the waist.

✓ Keep the bar close to your legs, skimming your thighs as you go down and up.

DIVA Troubleshooter

• **Why do I feel pain in my upper back?**

Check your alignment. You may be bending from the waist instead of from the hip joints. You may also be round-

"Concentration is the secret of strength."

Ralph Waldo Emerson

ing your back, which will cause pressure in the lower back and a strain in the upper back.

• Why can't I keep my knees straight?

You may not have developed enough flexibility in your hamstrings and/or your lower back. Only go down as far as you can with your knees straight. Also, make sure you initiate the motion by pushing your feet into the floor rather than pulling your arms up.

• The bar is too heavy for me.

If you need to, practice the movement with a light pole or a broomstick, then gradually move to using the bar. Evaluate whether or not the bar is really too heavy or if you're giving up because you're afraid. *Too heavy* means you can't do two repetitions with good technique. If you can perform two reps well, the bar is not too heavy. It's just heavy enough.

LUNGE

One day, my student Margo came to class reporting that her purse had been snatched on the subway the previous week. She described how a young man came up behind her, slit the shoulder strap with a box cutter, and made off with the bag.

"I *lunged* after him," she said, "and I practically tripped. By then he was gone."

"What do you mean when you say you *lunged*?" I asked.

"Huh?" Margo gave me a puzzled look. What a strange question. "You know . . . I tried to chase him."

There was nothing too unusual about Margo's experience. A man grabbed her purse, she instinctively started to chase him, and she tripped. Chasing purse snatchers in the subway isn't exactly a good idea whether you're stable on your feet or not. But Margo's story got me to thinking about the lunges we do in our workouts.

A lunge is a very basic human movement: the way we move assertively forward to protect ourselves or others or to give chase. Mothers of toddlers use the movement dozens of times a day to protect their curious children. Ballplayers use it to get a ball that is otherwise out of reach. And most of us have had the experience of lunging to catch a falling lamp or vase.

A lunge is strength in motion. It is a combination of being centered and planted firmly on the floor while moving forward. The lunge is a great exercise to learn because in life we're not always—or even usually—standing still.

Muscles Involved

Major: hips, buttocks, thighs and quadriceps, abdomen
Stabilizing: upper body

Most people think of a lunge as strictly a lower body exercise, but your upper body works as a stabilizing force, so all of your muscles are involved.

Benefits (Why You Do a Lunge)

➤ Tones and strengthens the hip, thigh, and gluteus muscles.
➤ Develops coordination and stability when you're in motion.
➤ Excellent strengthener for activities like Rollerblading, skiing, and tennis.

How to Do the Exercise

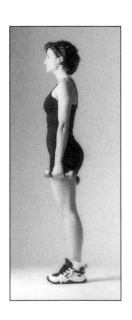 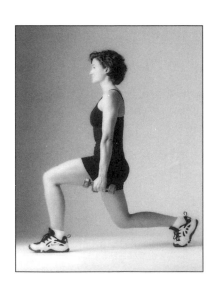 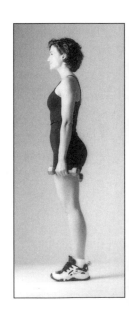

> ➤ Great alignment builder.
> ➤ Helps develop balance.

Position

1. Stand tall, lining up your joints: hips under shoulders, knees under hips, ankles under knees.
2. Place your feet parallel and hip width apart.
3. Pull in your navel.
4. Relax your shoulders and keep your arms close to your body.

Motion

1. Inhale. As you exhale, take a natural step forward with your left foot, keeping your chest lifted and your hips under your shoulders. Look straight ahead, not down.
2. With only about 20 percent of your weight on your left front foot, lower your body straight down until your right knee almost touches the floor. Don't allow your right knee to move beyond your toes. Hold this position long enough to maintain a straight body line.
3. Then, pulling your abs in, push your left foot into the floor, shifting your weight onto your left leg, and return to a standing position.
4. Repeat on the other side. Your goal is three sets of twenty repetitions.

ADVANCED: Add a bar or dumbbells. Hold the bar across the back of your shoulders. Hold the dumbbells at shoulder height. Add challenge by traveling across the floor with each step.

DIVA Secrets

✓ Instead of thinking of moving forward and backward, think of moving straight down and straight up. This will give you a good mental picture of maintaining your hips under your shoulders instead of leaning forward.

✓ Don't sit or squat when you are down in your lunge.

✓ Don't break at the waist.

✓ Don't look down. Look straight ahead.

✓ Don't stay in the lowered position too long—just long enough to secure yourself. Then come up quickly.

DIVA Troubleshooter

• **I feel myself leaning sideways and have a hard time maintaining a straight alignment.**

Check to see if your feet are in a hip-wide stance. If you don't leave enough space between your legs, it weakens your base of support, thereby interfering with your center of gravity. Next, check to see if your feet are far enough apart from front to back. A lunge should feel natural, not overextended. Finally, make sure that your hips are in line with your shoulder. Look in a mirror to check your form.

• **This exercise puts a strain on my knee.**

You may be twisting your knee slightly when you take a step or lunging too far forward. Your front knee should be in line with your front ankle. You may also be pushing into your toes, instead of distributing your weight evenly over your entire foot.

• **I have trouble coming back up without losing my form.**

Control the motion both ways—up and down—and work toward a moderate pace. If you perform the exercise too slowly, you'll spend too much time at the bottom and lose control coming back up; you begin wavering. Also, make sure you're wearing exercise shoes that have enough traction and support to hold you properly while you're doing this challenging exercise. Don't wear running shoes. They usually pitch your foot forward slightly.

• **My lower back feels stressed.**

You may not be engaging your abdominal muscles the correct way. Imagine that you're pulling your navel back toward your spine. This will give you the abdominal support you need. Keep your rib cage hinge closed.

"Be always sure you're right, then go ahead."

Davy Crockett

7

INTEGRITY

Integrity is the state of being entirely whole: physically, mentally, emotionally, and spiritually. Integrity is the inner voice of the DIVA, the steadying force that affirms your life just as it is.

We usually speak of integrity as a moral quality. When you say, "She has integrity," you mean that someone is honest, solid, unwavering in her convictions—and inherently trustworthy. We admire people with integrity above all others because we know they won't shift with the winds of opinion or fad. They're comfortable in their skin.

Learning integrity as a DIVA means establishing what feels right and what feels wrong for the essential *you*. If we're honest with ourselves, none of us can deny that it's a quality women have to work pretty hard to achieve.

Not long ago, I was having dinner with a friend, and the topic returned, as it often does, to her tales of woe about the man she lived with. Eileen and John had been together for almost eight years, and during that time I'm certain that Eileen shed a million tears. John was the kind of guy who couldn't give a woman a break. He picked at the way she dressed; he hated the way she wore her hair; he told her she was stupid because she liked to read mystery novels; he said her job was a dead end. You get the picture. Most of Eileen's women friends despised John, and we all urged her to leave him. He was toxic to her self-esteem. But Eileen always had a ready defense, no matter how hurtful John's behavior. She often said, "I know John really loves me."

Most women can relate to this: staying with a man who is taking daily nicks out of our very beings but denying that it's happening until the day we wake up and say, "What am I doing here?"

Integrity is knowing from the start whether a relationship is good for you because you know what you need and deserve. There's no doubt about it. No denial. It's all perfectly clear.

That's true in other areas of your life, as well. Can you picture what it would mean to really establish what feels right and what feels wrong for yourself? To know in your gut that you're doing the best you can for yourself? To know that your standards are the right ones for you to follow?

> **Write down your female role models for Integrity. Who are the secure ones?**

The exercises that represent Integrity focus on stability and balance. You may think you are balanced. After all, you walk around on two feet every day without falling down. But you might be surprised to learn how shaky your balance really is.

My client Karen was amazed at how unstable she was. "When I started doing the balancing exercises, I couldn't believe how hard they were," she admitted. "At first, I was very embarrassed. I thought, 'My God, I can't even stand up!' But I realized how little thought I had ever given to the question of balance and stability. It has so many practical ramifications. I remembered an incident that had happened a few months ago. I was walking down the street when suddenly a man came running out of a building and accidentally bumped into me. Before I knew what was happening, I was sprawled on the sidewalk in terrible pain from the cuts and bruises on my arms and legs. It took me several weeks to recover from this accident. I didn't even realize it at the time, but now I know that my problem was balance. People on the street could just push me over! I was determined to conquer this issue of bodily integrity, no matter how hard it was."

Karen felt humiliated when she had a hard time doing the Integrity exercises, but I told her that awareness comes from the practicing of being aware. If you've never had a reason to wonder if your leg was straight or if you were steady and centered, you wouldn't even know that you weren't steady and centered. That awareness is something you learn with practice. You don't just have it. The same goes for life. If you've never known how it feels to be secure and certain, you wouldn't necessarily know that you weren't.

The exercises that represent Integrity:

1. Cable balance
2. Step-up
3. Dumbbell Row
4. Abdominal integration

"For me, integrity means to maintain my physical well-being, and not to stray from my thinking of well-being. Not to get too involved in outside resources and distracted by other people. To stay centered and focused."
Sharon, 36

"I've started to feel my best when I am alone and am able to find happiness within myself. Eating well and exercising has increased my energy level and makes me feel great to be me—not someone else."
Tara, 32

"I feel stronger than ever that we as women do deserve to have our own personal goals. We need to continue to support and encourage each other, young and old, to be the rulers of our own lives, to build each other's self-worth, and not compete against each other, in all walks of our lives."
Cathy, 41

"I've learned that it is OK to be a klutz—you still deserve fitness. People are often told that they are not suited for athletics, so they haven't tapped that part of themselves. But there are many of us who will never be coordinated, and even for us, fitness and all of its benefits are within reach."
Peggy, 20

CABLE BALANCE

If you want to really improve your balance and sense of stability on the street, this exercise is a challenging and rewarding way to accomplish it.

Most of my students struggle with the cable balance. In fact, everyone hates it. It may be tedious and difficult at first, but the amazing thing is that you'll adapt very quickly, actually noticing improvement from set to set. Your body learns and remembers. It's a real victory when you can do one repetition perfectly. And when you're able to do ten or fifteen without holding onto anything, you'll be pretty proud of yourself. Although you never leave the ground, the sensation of grace and balance is as real as what a high-wire walker must feel when she moves along a wire, a hundred feet in the air. She's holding herself erect by the very force of her own body. And that's what you'll be doing, too.

Muscles Involved

Major: abdominals; calves; hamstrings; quadriceps; gluteus medius, maximus, minimus (in other words, your butt muscles)

Supporting: Every muscle. This isn't an isolation exercise where you're working one set of muscles. It's a balancing exercise, so you need every muscle group in your body to be doing its part, together.

Benefits (Why You Do the Cable Balance)

➤ Increases your body's stability in space.

➤ Improves your posture and balance.

➤ Strengthens and elongates your calves, ankles, and legs.

➤ Tones your whole body.

➤ Builds your agility and your appearance of confidence.

➤ Improves your coordination and action time.

You Will Need

➤ A rubber power band

➤ A flat 2" board or book

➤ A very heavy piece of furniture or a radiator to loop the band around

Position

1. Loop a rubber power band on a radiator, a firm table leg, or other very sturdy item.

2. Place one end of the rubber band around your left ankle so that the band crosses in front of the right foot.

3. Stand with both feet on the floor, with your right foot on a book that is flat and about one inch off the ground. Stand very straight, with both feet aligned and pointing forward.

4. Pull your abs in and your shoulders down.

5. Close your rib cage hinge.

Motion

1. Press the weight of your right leg into the book so that the left leg lifts slightly off the floor. Concentrate on keeping your hipbones straight. Don't hold onto anything. The key is to work on your balance.

2. Move your left foot slightly to the left, keeping both legs straight. Nothing should be moving but your left leg.

3. Repeat on the right side. At first, you'll have a hard time performing this exercise correctly more than two or three times. As you practice and gain balance, you will be able to do more repetitions. Your goal is three sets of ten repetitions.

How to Do the Exercise

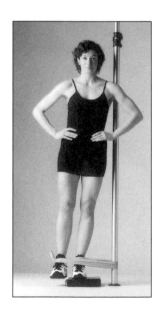 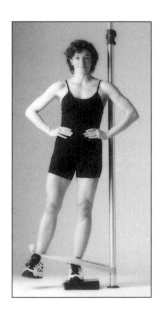 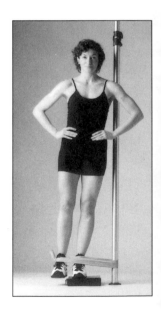

DIVA Secrets

✓ This exercise is an example of kinesthetic learning—slow and steady until the motion lives in your body. Don't be discouraged by slow progress. If you wobble and start to tip over, stop, regain your balance, and try again.

✓ Concentrate initially on how the exercise feels, not what it looks like. You should feel considerable tension along the outside of the thigh of your standing leg.

✓ This is a stabilizing exercise for your entire body.

✓ To achieve the correct alignment, think of keeping your rib cage raised above your hipbones.

✓ Keep your knees pointing straight ahead.

DIVA Troubleshooter

• How come I feel like I want to hold onto the wall?

This is common, but don't do it. If you hold on, you're just training yourself to do the exercise while holding on, which defeats the purpose of training for balance. You can't *balance* if you hold on. It's tedious, but stick with it. Take your time. Even one properly performed repetition is more effective than twenty repetitions performed while holding onto the wall.

• My foot tends to curl inward when I move it across the front. How do I keep it properly positioned?

Try not to pull with your foot. Contract the large muscles of your leg to begin the motion—not your foot. Keep your foot and toes facing forward throughout the exercise.

Don't give up.
"Sow an act and you reap a habit;
Sow a habit and you reap a character;
Sow a character and you reap a destiny."

Charles Reade

• How do I tell if my leg is straight?

If you don't have a mirror, think of extending your foot away from your body by pushing your weight into it. This should help you straighten both legs.

STEP-UP

The cable balance helped you stay grounded and balanced in a straight position. The step-up achieves the same thing in motion. My students also find this exercise surprisingly challenging. Although they walk up stairs every day of their lives, most of them admit that they automatically cling to a railing or place a hand against the wall for steadiness. For this reason, they don't get much sense of stability in motion.

Muscles Involved

Inner and outer thighs, hamstrings, buttocks

Since a step-up uses your body weight against gravity, it's very effective at tightening your butt without giving you bulky thighs.

Benefits (Why You Do a Step-Up)

➤ This exercise works the inner and outer thighs, shaping your leg in a balanced fashion.
➤ Develops your hamstrings in a lengthened manner, which aids in the appearance of a lifted butt.
➤ Improves your overall coordination.
➤ Aids in the development of muscle power.

You Will Need

➤ A sturdy bench, a commercial step unit, or the stair of a staircase.

Position

1. Stand straight in front of a sturdy bench, a commercial step unit, or the stair of a staircase.
2. Straighten your body, making sure your hips are aligned with your shoulders.
3. Pull your abs in and tuck your butt under.

Motion

1. Place your right foot on the bench. Line up your knee and ankle, then your knee and hip (do the same with the left leg). Think 90 degree angle.

How to Do the Exercise

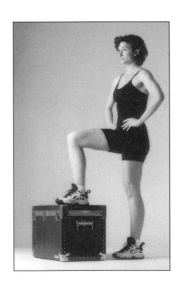
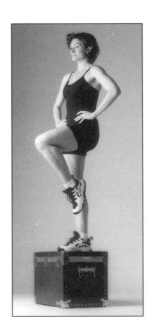
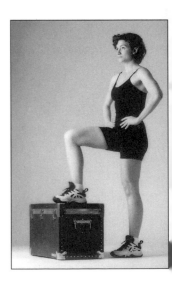

2. Inhale. As you exhale, start to shift your weight off your left foot by pushing your right foot into the bench. Simultaneously, roll your left foot off the floor to transfer your weight straight up.

3. Keep your hips and shoulders facing the front, and pull your navel in on the way up. Do not touch the bench with your left foot.

4. Hold the position until your balance is stable.

5. Step down.

6. Repeat on the same leg. Practice several times on each leg. Your goal is three sets of ten repetitions on each leg.

ADVANCED: Add five-pound dumbbells, holding them straight down along the sides of your body, without locking your elbows.
Gradually add weight and speed as your proficiency grows.

DIVA Secrets

✓ Keep your arms close to your body.

✓ Don't push off the leg that's on the floor. You'll know if you do because the exercise feels too easy.

✓ Straighten your leg all the way as you go up, without locking your knee.

✓ Watch out for the tendency to lean forward. Keep your hips straight under your shoulders.

✓ Don't break at the waist.

✓ Keep your head up, eyes forward.

✓ Your arms may go out in front of you for balance, but try to keep them in one position.

"Truth is the only safe ground to stand upon."
Elizabeth Cady Stanton,
The Woman's Bible

DIVA Troubleshooter

• Can I hold onto a railing at first, until I learn how to do it properly?

No, because doing it properly means learning to balance yourself as you travel through space. You can't learn to do this if you're holding on. It defeats the purpose of the exercise.

• This seems too easy. Am I doing something wrong?

If this exercise feels effortless at first, it probably means you are pushing off the bottom leg. When done correctly, there should be minimal stress on the standing leg; all of your weight should be transferred in a balanced motion onto the foot and leg that's on the bench.

• I feel wobbly and off-balance.

When you're a beginner, it may feel like you don't know how to push the active foot down into the bench. This will make you feel shaky on the way up. You'll feel your hamstrings and butt tighten as you get to the top. You'll also feel your inner and outer thighs struggle for the balance. That's normal.

• This exercise makes my knees hurt.

Do not let your knee get too far over your toe as you step up. Do not lock your knees to straighten your leg.

DUMBBELL ROW

It's probably not something you notice consciously, but as you go through the day, you perform many different kinds of movements. You're not always just standing and sitting straight. When you visualize the movement of a dumbbell row, think of it as sawing a piece of imaginary wood in a steady, relaxed rhythm.

Muscles Involved

Major: triceps, latissimus dorsi
Stabilizing: standing leg, entire torso, abdominal muscles

This may look like an arm exercise, since your arm is doing the movement, but it's really working the latissimus dorsi muscle that runs down the side of your upper body and your back. Your shoulder and arm are the hinge, not the main worker.

Benefits (Why You Do a Dumbbell Row)

➤ Builds muscle in your upper body.
➤ Aids alignment of your entire body, from knee to shoulder.
➤ Helps you learn to feel what's right and wrong when you use bending and lifting positions in everyday life.
➤ Helps you to stand up straight.
➤ Gives support to your rib cage.

You Will Need

➤ Two dumbbells: two or five pounds to start
➤ A bench

"Our nature lies in movement."
Pascal

Position

1. Place your left knee on the bench, using your left hand and arm to balance yourself.

2. Your right leg is bent slightly and placed firmly on the floor next to the bench.

3. Your right arm is hanging straight from your shoulder, holding the dumbbell. Be sure your body is properly held (look in a mirror to check your form). Your head and neck should be in alignment with your spine.

4. Pull your navel in, and close the rib cage hinge.

How to Do the Exercise

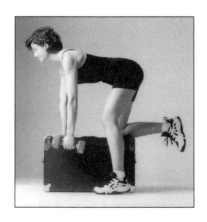 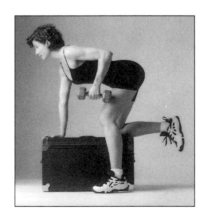 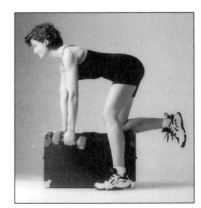

Motion

1. As if you were sawing a piece of imaginary wood, bring the dumbbell in a straight line back, so that your elbow is bent at the end of the motion. Exhale while you do.
2. While inhaling, return to the original position.
3. Perform the motion several times.
4. Repeat on the opposite side (right knee on the bench, left arm holding the weight).

ADVANCED: Add weight, but only when you can do it without changing your form. Increase the number of repetitions on each side.

DIVA Secrets

✓ Keep your back straight and steady to avoid strain.
✓ Pull your abs in to give you support.
✓ Keep thinking *alignment;* picture your body as one unit performing in sync.
✓ Don't forget to breathe.

DIVA Troubleshooter

• **This exercise hurts my lower back. I can't hold the leaning-over position.**

The temptation is to round your back and hunch over the bench—probably because that's the way you're used to leaning over. But you need to keep your back straight and aligned. You'll know you're out of alignment when your lower back aches.

• **I feel a strain in the knee of my standing leg.**

You're probably locking your knee. Always keep a slight bend in the knee.

• **Should I feel a strain in my latissimus dorsi?**

If you are doing the exercise correctly, you will feel a *stretch* in your lat muscles on the "down" part of the exercise. That's very different than a strain. A strain is an unnatural feeling of pain that makes you say "Ouch." That's a warning that you're not doing the exercise properly and may risk injury. Check your form.

ABDOMINAL INTEGRATION

Your abdominal muscles are the center of your being—the source of your spirit, your power, your identity. When you say, "I feel it in my *gut*," you're voicing a basic truth of human physiology. In effect, you're saying that everything evolves from the center of your being: action, emotion, will.

To be centered in life and in motion, your abdominal muscles must be strong. When you can feel the muscles in your abdominals, you experience a sense of power that seems almost mystical. You will begin to walk with the air of someone who matters in the world. Abdominal integration is the key to dignity.

On a practical level, your abdominals control the action of all of your muscles. Whenever you are doing an exercise, your abdominals are working. If they are weak, you will be weak. Have you ever watched the Korean martial art, tae kwon do? It's a good way to witness the centering of the body. The basic tae kwon do fighting position is a sturdy, bent-kneed stance, with all of the power coming from the center. A tae kwon do black belt can take any force, any punch to the stomach, and remain immovable. That's true whether it's a 100-pound woman or a 200-pound man. It's a demonstration that physical strength can sometimes be greater in a small person if her abdominal muscles are at their maximum level of fitness.

Can you imagine how you would feel if a mugger came up to you on the street and punched you as hard as he could in the stomach—and you remained steady? What a sensation of power there would be to know that no one could knock you down!

Of course, strengthening your abdominal muscles has other practical benefits for women, especially if you are of child-bearing age. If you are strong in the center, pregnancy can be easier and you can look forward to regaining a flat stomach after your baby is born. If you've already had children and your abdomen is weak, you can still get back to the youthful body you once had, although it may take a bit more work. I've even worked with women who had cesarean sections, which means their abdominal muscles were sliced open. Some of them have never been able to achieve a flat stomach, no matter how hard they worked, because they couldn't feel their muscles. With time and consistency, these women have been able to work through their weakness; and while they might not be able to achieve the perfect flat stomach of their youth (at least, without plastic surgery), they look and feel stronger and more fit than they ever could have imagined.

Muscles Involved

Abdomen, rib cage, buttocks

Benefits (Why You Do Abdominals)

➤ Builds a strong, flat stomach.
➤ Reduces lower back problems by creating a balance between your abdominal and lower back muscles.
➤ Improves your posture by lifting your center and straightening your back.
➤ Protects you against injury and strain when you're lifting or carrying something heavy.
➤ Enables you to do every other exercise.

➤ Enables you to have a healthier pregnancy, an easier labor, and quickly return to shape after your baby is born.

You Will Need

➤ A mat on the floor

Position

1. Lie on the floor, faceup, with your knees bent and hip-width apart.
2. Plant your feet firmly on the floor, a comfortable distance from your buttocks.
3. Make sure you can feel your entire back against the floor.
4. Cup your hands lightly against the backs of your ears or your head.
5. Pull your navel down, breathing out, while your feet press gently into the floor.

How to Do the Exercise

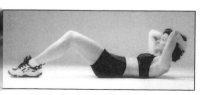 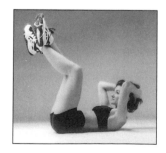 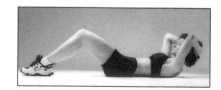

*"There can be no real freedom with-
out the freedom to fail."*

Eric Hoffer

Motion

1. Take a deep breath. As you exhale, pull your rib cage down and raise your shoulders slightly from the floor, keeping your back flat and your eyes toward the ceiling. (You are being raised by your abdominal muscles, not your head and neck.) Keep your rib cage hinge closed, your navel pushing down.

2. As you inhale, release back slowly to the floor, controlling the motion on the way down (don't flop).

3. Repeat four times, rest, and check to make sure you aren't feeling tension in your neck; then repeat four more times. Your goal, with more practice, is three sets of twenty repetitions.

ADVANCED VARIATIONS: Perform the same movement with your arms stretched so that your fingers reach for the ceiling. Be sure you're raising up with your abdominals, not pulling with your arms.

Cross your ankles and lift your legs in the air. Perform the same movement. Line up your knees with your hips.

As if someone were pulling your buttocks under with a string, slightly pull them up and off the floor, using your abdominal muscles.

DIVA Secrets

✓ When you're just starting out, it may be hard to raise your-self using your abdominal muscles because they're still weak. Don't worry about going up very far. Even the slightest raising is effective.

✓ Beware the temptation to pull yourself up using the neck

and shoulders. Your hands should be relaxed lightly, not hanging on. Your head is still, with your eyes fixed on the ceiling.

✓ Keep checking to be sure you can feel your entire back against the floor. This will prevent back strain.

DIVA Troubleshooter

• **I feel a lot of strain in my neck.**

If you're using your abdominal muscles, you won't feel a strain in your neck. This is a sign that you're pulling up head first, straining the back of your neck. Keep your head and neck still by focusing your eyes straight ahead.

• **My lower back aches.**

Pull your navel down to help your lower back make contact with the floor. The key to keeping your back on the floor is to practice the rib cage hinge.

• **How far am I supposed to raise myself off the floor?**

Don't worry about raising yourself very much at first. Concentrate on pulling down from the middle of your body. Your abdominals will be engaged and have to work just as hard when the movement is small. The height of your shoulders off the floor will increase with your abdominal strength and the flexibility of your back.

• **I can't feel my abdominal muscles. How do I know if they're working?**

Place your hand on your navel as you do the exercise. If

your navel goes *down* while your shoulders go *up*, your abs are working.

• Can I do abdominal exercises during my menstrual period?

That's up to you. They won't hurt you. But if you suffer from cramps or your flow is heavy, you might be uncomfortable. Listen to your body; it will tell you whether it needs rest or movement.

• Can I do abdominal exercises when I'm pregnant?

Most healthy pregnant women are encouraged to exercise, but always check with your doctor first. You should be able to continue normal abdominal work during your first trimester. After that, you may need to modify them so you're not lying flat on the floor. When you're lying flat, your baby presses against the vein that supplies blood to your heart. The result is dizzines and extreme discomfort. But there are many ways you can work your abdominal muscles without lying down. Here's one great example.

ABDOMINAL EXERCISE FOR PREGNANT WOMEN

- Stand straight in the center of the floor, with your spine lengthened and your head straight and focused forward. Place your feet together at the heels in a V. (You might recognize this position as a basic ballet plié.)
- Take a deep breath. Keeping your feet together and your body straight, bend your knees as much as feels comfortable on the exhale. (It doesn't matter if you bend your knees a little or a lot, so don't overdo it.)
- As you come back up, imagine that a cord is pulling your abdominal muscles in and your navel to the back of your spine. Squeeze your butt at the same time.
- This exercise works other muscles besides the abdominal muscles: in particular, your butt, quads, and inner thighs.

8

VITALITY

Vitality is energy. It is the quality that distinguishes the living from the nonliving. There is a huge difference between *participating* in your life and just watching other people with the hope that their luck, beauty, brains, or strength will rub off on you. Women who possess the quality of vitality take risks. They pick themselves up when they fall. They're not easily discouraged.

One of the most inspiring examples of vitality I've seen in my work came from a woman who was quite obese. Marsha weighed 250 pounds, and she seemed to be the opposite of vitality when she began to work with me at the insistence of her doctor. I was touched by her commitment to change, though. She said, "I'm tired of just watching my life pass by and seeing everyone else get to do things I can't. I want to live, too."

Marsha couldn't imagine performing the simple movements that most people take for granted—like walking up stairs, jumping over a mud puddle, or running for a bus. She was exhausted by exertion of any kind. It was an exhaustion of the spirit as well as the body, because she was so discouraged.

In spite of how far Marsha had to go, she stayed with the program, four days a week. She worked through pain and stress, and she felt more optimistic even before she could see any results. Vitality became a living thing inside her.

Today, two and a half years after Marsha started working out, she weighs 170 pounds. She still thinks she has a way to go in that regard, but some of that weight is solid muscle now, instead of fat. She looks great because she feels great and moves with confidence. Marsha took a chance on her life, and it paid off.

The foundation of vitality lies in developing courage. Courage is the quality that gives you the guts to try what's new and different. It helps you transcend your fears. With courage, you plunge into the darkness, not knowing what you'll find. You give yourself the chance to live the experience of doing. That's the difference between living and nonliving.

When you're working out, vitality means being totally present for the exercise you're doing. Focus. Put everything else aside. Resolve to carve out time *mentally* as well as physically. Enjoy the gift of movement. Force yourself to pay attention to yourself—something women have a hard time doing. Think, "I deserve this for *me*."

Concentrate on what you feel when you're doing the exercise. Get in a zone. Feeling is an important part of training. You need to *feel* what is the right way and the wrong way. This is another kinesthetic aspect of the training process. Feeling isn't about thinking. It's about being there.

This is a total mind-body system, so pay attention to your emotions. It's normal to sometimes feel good and sometimes feel full of self-doubt. You might have times when you get discouraged and say, "Who do I think I'm kidding? I can't do this."

You may feel that way because you're used to hearing it from other people. There are always going to be people in your life who are negative reinforcers. Think of this as giving yourself something you have a hard time getting from other people. (By the way, people act like they just discovered the mind-body connection. But how could it be any other way? Exertion demands a mind-body connection.)

Ask yourself, "How do I want to be?" Then, be it. Know that "being it" isn't some far-off, abstract goal. It starts the minute you make the commitment. "Being it" begins with doing, acting, breathing, seeing the very way you want to be. Choose your favorite active role model or female athlete. Consider how she organizes her life. Start there: How does she train? How does she eat? And so on. Then, see if anything makes sense for your life and try it. Adjust it and make it *yours*. When you begin to ask these questions and to search out the answers, your quest will lead you in the right direction. Then you'll find that some things will work for you and others won't. It's all part of learning to define yourself—in your own time and in your own way. Trial and error and experience are the best teachers in the world.

> **Write down your female role models for Vitality. Who are the courageous ones?**

You'll discover that learning to focus during your training will help you focus in other areas of your life. You'll find yourself being able to make decisions faster, to cut to the chase and move past all of the extraneous matter.

Research is all well and good, and reading up on things makes you smarter, but you must practice while you learn and

"Being physically fit has increased my energy, stamina, and confidence. That's what I call vitality. I walk down the street a little cockier now and feel a little more assured inside. Being physically strong has led me to be more mentally strong."

Peggy, 20

"I'm beginning to know what it means to feel joyful about living each day. I have always been one to dwell on the things I didn't like about myself, other people, or my job. Now I think, 'Why am I wasting my wonderful life on gloominess?' I want to experience life as wonderful."

Cathy, 41

"I have more energy, more confidence. Setting small goals and achieving them has really helped me be happy, centered, at peace. My attitude and behavior have definitely improved. I love seeing the results of my hard work: new muscles, increasing weights. It has also helped me attack hard projects with more vigor."

Lynn, 33

put it into action. Knowledge is meaningless unless you use it. Potential is nothing unless you realize it. Internalize the knowledge to gain a physical understanding of what you're doing. That means getting off your butt and sweating. No ifs, ands, or buts about it.

The exercises that represent Vitality:

1. Squats
2. Vertical jumps
3. Side-to-side jumps
4. Aerobics (cardiovascular activity)

SQUAT

Squatting is a natural, primal activity. It symbolizes getting close to the earth—engaging intimately with nature. Like all of the exercises in the DIVA System, it is not superimposed or phony. It's what you really do in life.

The best way to visualize a squat is to think about what you do when you sit down in a chair. You lead with your butt. Begin by practicing sitting in a chair and standing up. Do this several times to become familiar with the motion. Now you're ready to do the actual squat.

Muscles Involved

Buttocks (gluteal muscles), hamstrings, quadriceps, calves, abdominals, upper and lower back

Benefits (Why You Do a Squat)

➤ It's a foundation for one of your most common actions: standing and sitting.
➤ It gives you a tighter butt.
➤ It strengthens your hamstrings.
➤ It builds the stamina and coordination you need to jump.

Position

1. Stand with your legs hip width apart. Your feet and knees should be in a parallel position.
2. Be sure your feet are flat on the floor. Push your feet into the floor.

3. Keep your chest high.

4. You may hold your arms away from you for balance or keep them close to your body.

Motion

1. Sit straight down, leading with your butt. Make sure you're doing a sitting motion, not bending over from the waist. Your thighs should be parallel to the floor.

2. Come up as you exhale, pulling your abdominal muscles in and pushing your heels down. Straighten your legs but don't lock or jam your knees.

How to Do the Exercise

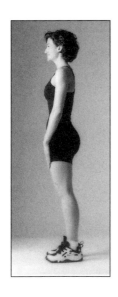 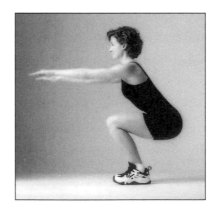 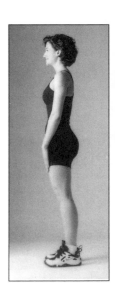

3. Repeat six times, then do six more. Your goal is three sets of fifteen repetitions.

> ADVANCED: Add a bar, holding it across your shoulders, with your fingers facing forward. Or add a set of dumbbells, holding them at shoulder level.

DIVA Secrets

✓ To get the sensation of planting your feet firmly, pretend your feet are your hands, spread out and pushed down against the floor.

✓ Push your feet down and pull your abs in as you are standing.

✓ Don't look down. Look straight ahead.

✓ Be sure to keep your back straight. This exercise is about moving from the hip joint, not bending forward from the waist.

✓ If you use a bar, you will have to get used to the feeling of having a bar on your shoulders. Your tendency will be to push forward to accommodate the weight. Concentrate on keeping your form. (Don't use a bar or dumbbells until you have the exercise down pat.)

DIVA Troubleshooter

• Why do I fall forward?

You're bending over. Remember: Your body goes where your head goes. Keep your chest lifted. Don't break at the waist. When you sit down, bend at the hip joints where your legs connect to your body.

• I have trouble understanding the position.

Take a regular chair and practice sitting down and getting up, over and over. Pay attention to the movement and the action of the muscles. It's exactly like that.

• My back hurts. What am I doing wrong?

You're not using your abdominal muscles to support your lower back. Check to see that your rib cage hinge is closed and that your navel is pulled in. Look in the mirror sideways. If your lower back is arched, you're in the wrong position.

• I feel a strain in my neck when I use a bar.

You may have the bar placed too high on your neck. The bar should be resting lightly across the back of your trapezius muscles across the top of your back and below your shoulders. Make sure that your arms are supporting the bar as well—it's what makes the squat a total body exercise.

• I have trouble getting my heels all the way down on the floor.

This is a common problem for people who have tight achilles tendons. Place a one-inch-thick book or piece of wood under your heels. This should help keep your heels down.

VERTICAL JUMP

A jump is a squat that moves. Why jump? There are some compelling reasons. First, the motion of jumping is symbolic of overcoming hurdles in your life. You can actually feel the exhilaration flowing through your body. You may recall a time, when you were very young, when you jumped rope for hours on end. Jumping exercises will enable you to bring that spirited young girl back into the world. Jumping also develops plyometric power—which is your "springing" power. You'll learn to move faster and more explosively. Another advantage is that jumping raises your heart rate and uses more calories in less time.

Allow yourself to be a beginner, even if you feel a little silly. Take the time to learn. Jumping equals vitality. Get the feeling of exuberance.

Jumping is a skill you may not think you need, but once you can do it, it changes everything. Think of it as trusting your body to move through space and feel the childlike joy of letting go. It's never too late to experience joy.

Muscles Involved

This exercise uses almost every muscle: abdominals, legs, calves, back, shoulders.

Benefits (Why You Do Vertical Jumps)

➤ Develops agility.
➤ Builds muscle definition.
➤ Develops speed. The faster you are, the better your reaction time.

ANAEROBIC POWER

This is an anaerobic exercise. Anaerobic power is being able to do brief spurts of motion, which is then followed by recovery time to allow your body to replenish its oxygen stores. Three minutes is a long time, so you'll want to do very short periods of activity, then rest. The difference between aerobic and anaerobic exercise is the difference between having enough oxygen and not having enough oxygen. (Aerobic means *with oxygen;* anaerobic means *without oxygen.*) Anaerobic exercises are explosive, fast motions, like sprints, jumps, or anything that requires short bursts of energy.

➤ Eliminates fear of moving through space.

➤ Gives you anaerobic power.

➤ It's fun!

You Will Need

➤ A low platform, a sturdy low bench, or a bar on the floor

Position

1. Stand straight, about two to four inches in front of the center of the bench or bar, with your feet together.
2. Squat down.

How to Do the Exercise

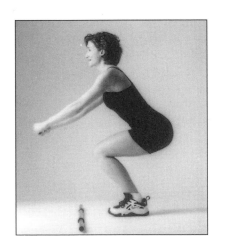
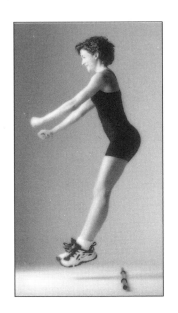
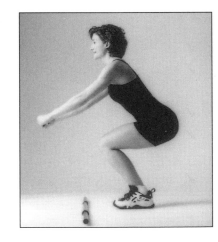

3. Make sure your shoulders are down.
4. Hang your arms loose by your sides.

Motion

1. Inhale as you squat low, like you were sitting down in a chair, and extend your arms behind you.
2. Exhale as you jump onto the platform or over the bar, swinging your arms upward to propel the motion.
3. Land toes first and instantly roll your weight through your feet to your heels. Think "toe, ball, heel." Keep your knees bent.
4. Practice several times, working on letting your feet land together. Your goal is three sets of fifteen repetitions.

ADVANCED: Add weights, holding them close to your body for stability. Or add risers to your bench and jump higher.

DIVA Secrets

✓ Jump straight up, not forward.
✓ In the beginning stages, use your arms to help launch your body.
✓ Don't land with a flat foot. (See sidebar).
✓ Inhale as you marshall your forces; exhale as you leap into the air.
✓ Keep your eyes straight ahead while maintaining the bench within your sight range. Do this without looking down; your body goes where your head goes.

FOOT FLEXES

You can practice for the landing motion by doing foot flexes, which help to strengthen your feet. Most people don't realize that their feet and ankles need to be stretched and strengthened, just like the other joints and muscles. Foot flexes help you to roll through your feet. This means you'll be using your feet to cushion the impact instead of just pounding into the floor. You'll prevent injury and sustain your athletic life longer. To do a foot flex:

1. *Sit on the floor and place your rubber band around the ball of your foot.*
2. *Holding the band tense in both hands, flex your foot and hold.*
3. *Then point your toe, creating resistance against the band.*
4. *Repeat.*

"Every great and commanding movement in the annals of the world is the triumph of enthusiasm."
Ralph Waldo Emerson

DIVA Troubleshooter

• **I have trouble getting both of my feet to land together.**

Practice your foot flexes to learn the motion of rolling through your feet. Remember that jumping also requires coordination, and that takes time to develop. Don't jump until you have practiced step-ups and squats.

• **I'm afraid of tripping.**

Start low—even with a line on the floor—and add height in small increments as you get comfortable.

• **How do I come down from the bench?**

Step off the bench or platform one foot at a time. Don't *jump* down from the bench.

SIDE-TO-SIDE JUMPS

Side-to-side, or lateral, jumps are for balance, coordination, power, speed, agility, and reaction time. It's important to learn how to move your feet, which is the most natural motion in the world.

This exercise is neuromuscular, which means you're training your nervous system to respond faster. The muscles in your back, chest, and shoulders are stabilized. It is also an anaerobic exercise, meaning it uses short bursts of energy. That translates into making you faster, increasing your lung capacity, and achieving more efficient energy production. This means you're beginning to compound one system on top of another. Your skills are increasing.

Muscles Involved

Calves, feet, hamstrings, quadriceps, butt, abs

Benefits (Why You Do This Exercise)

➤ Helps you be more coordinated.
➤ Increases your stability in a lateral motion.
➤ Strengthens your anaerobic power.
➤ Strengthens your inner and outer thighs.
➤ Great practice for winter skiing.

You Will Need

➤ A bar on the floor

Position

1. Stand straight next to the right-hand center of the bar.
2. Slightly bend your knees.
3. Keep your feet together and firmly planted on the floor.
4. Pull your abs in, and squat slightly.
5. Tuck your elbows into your sides.

Motion

1. Inhale. On the exhale, jump sideways in one motion, keeping your elbows in and your upper body still. Your entire body should be facing forward.

How to Do the Exercise:

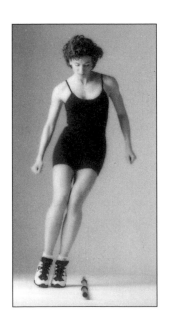 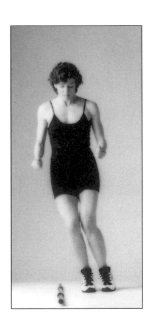 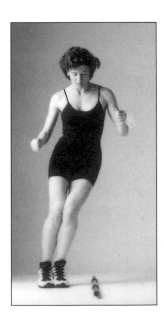

2. Keep your thighs together and your hamstrings active.
3. Land in a rolling motion on your feet: toe, ball, and heel.
4. Repeat the same motion back, and continue jumping side to side. Your goal is three sets of fifteen repetitions.

VARIATION: FRONT AND BACK JUMP: Stand facing the bar with your body in the tightly controlled skiing position described above.

Jump forward on the exhale. Immediately repeat the motion backward.

ADVANCED VARIATIONS: Increase your speed, using a stopwatch.

Jump while holding 3-5 pound dumbbells.

Jump on one foot.

DIVA Secrets

✓ Beginners: To practice, start with a crack in the floor, then add a broomstick, and finally a bench.

✓ Think of it like a skiing motion or a gentle springing.

✓ Keep your hips and shoulders in the same line, facing forward.

✓ Keep your upper body stable by holding your arms close to your body.

✓ Make sure there is give in your knees.

✓ If the idea of jumping scares you or feels awkward, begin by practicing squats, then vertical jumps, until you're comfortable with the motion.

✓ If you're doing the exercise correctly, you'll feel it in your butt, hamstrings, and calves.

"Grace is the absence of everything that indicates pain, or difficulty, hesitation or incongruity."

Wiliam Hazlett

DIVA Troubleshooter

• I feel a jarring sensation when I make impact.

You're landing flat on your feet. Practice your foot flexes until you master the rolling foot motion.

• My ankles twist when I land. I can't keep them straight.

You're jumping too soon. Work on your balance by practicing the cable balance exercise on page 78 in the Integrity section.

• I feel a strain in my hips.

You're probably twisting your body to follow the movement instead of keeping your hips and shoulders lined up and facing forward. Remember, your whole body is moving sideways in a single motion.

• I have pain in my knees.

If you have knee pain, you're not using your feet to soften the landing or you're landing with straight legs. Make sure your feet transfer the impact by landing through the toes and rolling back. Practice the foot flex exercise shown on page 109. Also, make sure you've practiced all the exercises to prepare your muscles properly.

• How do I compensate for high arches?

The best way to compensate for high arches is to strengthen your feet, using the foot flexes. If that doesn't help, you may need arch supports on your shoes. Check with an orthopedist before you jump on a regular basis.

• When I jump, I feel a strain in my lower back.

If you feel back pain, you're not using your abdominal muscles to support your back. Practice doing squats, paying special attention to the abdominal involvement. Make sure the rib cage hinge is closed while you are in motion.

AEROBICS

I've been teaching aerobics classes for the past fifteen years, usually in those packed, sweaty classes you see in gyms and fitness clubs. Many people find the very idea of engaging in this form of mass torture ridiculous. As one woman with a high-pressure job said, quite reasonably, "I work a very stressful ten-hour day, and then I'm supposed to put myself through this and get even more exhausted before I drag myself home and fall into bed? You call that a life?"

No, not really. (Although, I wonder if aerobics is the problem here.) I think it's time we put aerobics into perspective.

First of all, doing aerobic activity doesn't mean joining an aerobics class—unless, of course, you want to. You can achieve aerobic fitness without ever breathing the steamy air of a gym.

Second, aerobic power is a basic human requirement for cardiovascular health, overall fitness, and a lean body. Many thousands of years ago, long before the word *aerobic* was ever coined, our ancestors lived in a highly aerobic state. They ran to catch and kill their food. They traveled hundreds of miles on foot to procure more food. They were the ultimate example of a lean, mean, fighting machine. They used their bodies as they were meant to be used, as a tool for survival.

Our modern life is pretty far away from that. We don't climb stairs; we take elevators. We don't walk; we drive cars or take trains. We don't chase down our food; we pick it up in the supermarket at our leisure. Most of us don't even perform demanding physical labor; we work in offices with the air-conditioning running full blast. God forbid we should sweat!

What is the result of this splendid modern existence? Cardiovascular disease is the number-one killer of both men and women. Obesity is a national disgrace. Most people couldn't comfortably walk up a hill, much less run for their lives.

Achieving aerobic capacity is the number-one way to reverse all of these conditions. It is the very essence of Vitality.

Here's the way aerobic exercise works. Unlike anaerobic activity (which we experienced with jumps), aerobic activity is a longer, repetitive motion that you perform until your heart rate reaches a certain level. Your breathing action sucks in oxygen and delivers it to your muscles to keep them going.

Now, let's talk about how we're going to learn to be aerobic. Later, I'll introduce you to some great aerobic activities that are fun, exhilarating, and can be performed outside your four walls. But first, let's get the idea down by practicing a couple of basic aerobic movements and getting a sense of how they feel.

Muscles Involved

Your whole body is involved in aerobic activity. Every muscle is working to full capacity—especially your heart muscle.

Benefits (Why You Do Aerobics)

➤ It's a primary factor in cardiovascular health and overall fitness.
➤ Aerobic activity will help strengthen your bones and add flexibility to your joints—a big issue for women, because we're susceptible to osteoporosis in later life.
➤ It's the best way to lose weight. Aerobic activity expends more energy than any other workout.
➤ Gives you real control of your body—a sense of confidence that you can move fast without getting injured or falling down.

FINDING YOUR TARGET HEART RATE ZONE

The best way to be sure you have reached an aerobic level is to check your heart rate. Every person has a zone at which their hearts are pumping aerobically. The lower end of the zone is less exertion; the higher rate is more exertion. If you're a beginner, stay at the lower end and slowly add more time and intensity until you've built up your endurance.

To calculate your approximate heart rate zone, subtract your age from 220. That number is an estimate of your 100 percent heart rate. To find your zone, multiply that number by .85. Don't go higher than that. Then, multiply the original number by .60. Below that, you won't be working aerobically.

Example: a thirty-year-old woman:

$$220 - 30 = 190$$
$$190 \times .85 = 162$$
$$190 \times .60 = 114$$

You'll want to work within this range.

An easy way to check your pulse while you're exercising is to press your fingers against the pulse at your wrist. Count the number of beats you feel in 6 seconds and multiply it by 10. This is not an exact measure, but it's close enough to give you an estimate.

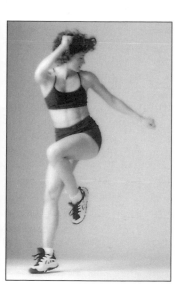

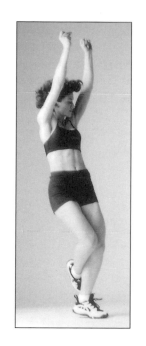

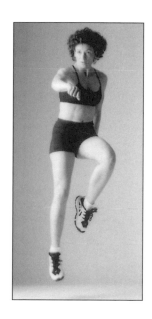

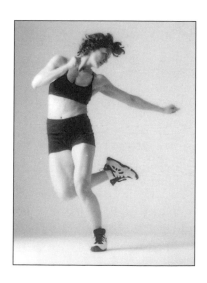

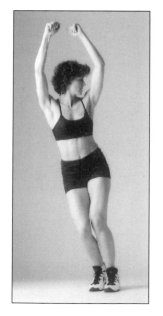

> ➤ Boosts your energy for the whole day.

> ➤ Provides a life skill that you can use whenever you have to move fast.

A Sample Aerobic Exercise

Position

1. First, perform the warm-up and stretching exercises described in the Aspiration section on pages 126–131. This will get your body loose and stretched.
2. Stand straight (but not rigid) with your arms to your side and your feet slightly apart.
3. Close your rib cage hinge.

Motion

A NOTE: Although it normally takes at least twenty minutes of steady movement to achieve aerobic capacity, in the beginning, you might have trouble doing the following exercise at its full length and pace. Begin by practicing for as long as you can and at whatever pace allows you to keep moving.

1. Take a deep breath. As you exhale, move your left leg out a bit past your shoulders.
2. Move your right leg so that your toe touches the center of your left foot. Keep breathing in rhythm.
3. Move your right leg out a bit past your shoulders, then bring your left leg in so that your toe touches the center of your right foot. It's an easy side-to-side motion, kind of like a dance step.

4. Start slowly and gradually increase your speed. Play music if it will help you get into the motion.

5. After three minutes, engage your upper body by lightly swinging your arms across the front of your body in sync with your leg movements.

6. After three more minutes, and without slowing down, begin doing a marching motion with your legs, bringing your knees up as high as possible. Bend your arms and begin moving them back and forth in sync with the marching.

7. After three minutes, again without stopping, return to the original movement. Keep going for three minutes.

8. Now, without changing your speed, begin a step-together-step movement across the floor to your left for as much room as you have; then reverse and go the other way. Continue for fifteen minutes.

9. Finally, put it all together: side-to-side, march, step-together-step. Repeat the sequence for three minutes.

10. At the end, don't just stop. Gradually slow down, stretching your arms. You should be breathing pretty hard and are probably wet with perspiration. Congratulations! That's the whole idea.

DIVA Secrets

✓ Keep your eyes off the clock. The seconds and minutes will crawl. Psychologically, you'll feel that it's impossible. Instead, play music or watch the view. (Some people find aerobics their best thinking time.)

✓ A clue that you're getting in the aerobic zone is that you break out in a sweat. It's the natural way your body cools down.

> *REAL-LIFE ALTERNATIVES*
>
> So many activities have aerobic capabilities that your options are endless. Here are a few of the best for a good workout and weight loss. Choose those that fit you. Make it fun!
>
> JUMP ROPE: Feet together; increments of 2, 4, 6, and then 10 minutes
>
> BRISK WALKING: Nonstop walking at a pace of about one mile every fifteen minutes. Go at least three miles.
>
> JOGGING OR RUNNING: Nonstop at a comfortable speed. Continue for a minimum of twenty minutes. Keep increasing your duration and speed.
>
> BICYCLING: Continue for thirty minutes without stopping. Don't rest on your shoulders. Make it active. When you're ready, incorporate hills.
>
> FORMULATED AEROBIC WORKOUTS: If you prefer, join an aerobics class or use aerobics videotapes. Check out your instructors to be sure they're authorized, experienced, and encourage correct form.
>
> AT THE GYM: Besides aerobics classes, you can do thirty minutes on the treadmill, stationary bike, step machine, rowing machine, or ski machine. All provide excellent, safe workouts.

✓ Stay loose. Don't get uptight about doing aerobics. It's the same as dancing and other fun activities. Remember when you were a kid and could jump rope for hours or play volleyball for an entire afternoon? Recapture that youthful energy.

✓ Look for opportunities to get aerobic in your day-to-day life. Walk to work. Bike to work. Climb the stairs instead of taking the elevator. (It won't wear you out. It will boost your energy.)

✓ Before you engage in an aerobics program, check with your doctor, especially if you have any conditions that might be affected (high blood pressure, heart problems, pregnancy, a bad back, etc.).

"Remember that nobody will ever get ahead of you as long as he is kicking you in the seat of the pants."
Walter Winchell

DIVA Troubleshooter

• **I run out of breath after about six minutes. Should I stop?**

If you're not used to doing aerobics, it's going to feel unnatural and overly strenuous. Assuming your doctor has given the go-ahead, you should try to continue. One trick is to slow down without stopping, then speed up again when you catch your breath. Be sure you're breathing deeply throughout. You need oxygen to do this. And take it slowly. You don't have to work up to your maximum heart rate.

• **My arms feel tired and slightly strained after an aerobic exercise.**

Good! This should let you know that you're using all your muscles. Once your body gets used to the motion, your arms will feel less tired.

• **Whenever I begin to really get going, I get a terrible cramp in my side.**

You're probably not getting enough oxygen. Be sure you're taking full breaths. If you do get a cramp, try not to stop. Sometimes it helps to raise your arm above your head to release the cramp. Or slow down a little. But keep breathing!

• **How will I know when I'm ready for a more strenuous aerobic activity?**

You'll know. Your body will get impatient. It will demand more exertion to make you sweat. You'll feel bored and restless. Use your heart rate as a guide.

• **Can I do aerobics if I'm pregnant?**

Absolutely (as long as your doctor gives the go-ahead). Many women exercise aerobically right up to the day of delivery. It keeps you fit and helps you with the heavy breathing you need for labor. Try to stick to low-impact aerobics (like walking instead of running). Drink plenty of water, and carefully monitor your heart rate.

9

ASPIRATION

Aspiration is having a belief in the future, a willingness to dream and experiment and incorporate your dreams, expectations, and commitments into a life plan. Think of it this way:

Determination is what gets you there.
Integrity helps you do it in a way that feels right.
Vitality gives you the energy you need to perform.
Aspiration is living it, formulating your dreams and moving
toward the future.

Aspiration requires a belief in yourself. It means being in the space of success before you've even started.

> **Write down your role models for Aspiration.**
> **Who are the women of hope?**

Aspiration is not grim. It isn't an obsessive focus on your goals. If anything, having aspiration gives you joy, flexibility, and pleasure.

"Aspiration is taking the dedication and determination that you know you possess and applying it to the place in your life where it is missing. I finally got brave enough to do that with my writing, and you know what? I'm a real writer now, not just an insecure dabbler."

Joan, 26

....

"For me, aspiration is knowing that the mind, body, and soul are connected—and they all have to be nurtured equally and at the same time. When I learned to find my soul in physical activity, I was a new person."

Amy, 31

....

"Aspiration is the acceptance of and respect for your body. It's appreciating differences and knowing that the world would be very boring if everyone looked the same."

Fran, 38

The dreams that you dream, the hopes that you hold dearly, the goals that you aspire to are not really about fitness. They're about having a rich and fulfilling life.

In the Aspiration section, we're going to start putting it all together, just like you'll do in real life. In addition to the actual exercises, there are other things you'll do during a workout that make it complete, and without which it won't be effective or safe. You may already know about them. But if you're a beginner, by now you're probably wondering exactly how you start putting all the various pieces together. Well, for one thing, you don't just grab a weight and begin. Let's go through a typical forty-minute workout. It may take you more time. The best thing to do is follow the instructions, and don't think about time. Once you get used to the rhythm, you can judge how long each step takes. Make your own adjustments for time. I'll talk you through the routine now, so when you start your Progression One workout in the next section, you'll know just what to do.

Before you begin, write the date, time, and workout details in your journal. You can call this the Practice Workout.

Warm-Up: Five to Eight Minutes

Your workout imitates life. Think about it. You probably don't just jump out of bed in the morning and head for work. You get dressed, maybe relax over breakfast, watch the news. You mentally and physically get ready for your day. Well, your body needs to get ready, too, if you plan to work it. You can't just put on your workout clothes and start lifting weights. First, you have to let your body know that you're going to be active. You have to nudge your heart into action and raise your heart rate so it's set to perform the exercises. It's also a way to prevent injury. You can't stretch tight muscles. They have to be loose and flexible. That's the purpose of a warm-up. The warm-up also helps you put your head in a physical mindset.

A warm-up consists of five or ten minutes of light aerobic exercise. You can do part of the aerobic routine I laid out in the Vitality section, or you can improvise: Walk for half a mile; jump rope for a few minutes; put on music and do your favorite dance step. If you're at a gym or have home equipment, do five minutes on a stationary bike or a rowing machine. But keep it light. You only want to break a sweat.

Some people think the warm-up is just stretching. But if you really analyze the way your muscles work, you'll realize that it's hard to stretch tight or cold muscles. For an image, think of taffy. When it's hard, you can't pull it. But once it gets warm and pliable, you can.

Stretching is the second step, after you've warmed up.

Stretch: Five to Seven Minutes

The beginning stretch is called, appropriately, the Good Morning, Sunshine stretch. It's a real feel-good stretch, and it even works on rainy, gray days.

1. Stand tall. Open your legs to a nice wide stance—a little beyond your shoulders but not so wide that you feel unbalanced. Your shoulders are dropped and relaxed (but not slumped). Your neck is long, eyes straight ahead.

2. Open your hands, palms turned up toward the sky. Spread your fingers wide.

3. As you inhale deeply, slowly raise and open your arms outward from your body, and lift your head toward the

"For me, aspiration is discarding the ludicrous physical and emotional ideals that are forced upon women—not just by men, but by other women, too. We are taught at an early age that we must succeed in very particular ways (being pretty, slender, financially successful) and if girls are taught that it's OK to be who they are, not who we want them to be, then they will be far more well-adjusted than their predecessors. In that vein, boys should be taught that it's not just external beauty that makes a woman attractive. As for our generation, I think that choosing a personal mantra such as 'I am a worthy individual' or 'I am beautiful because of who I am,' is an invaluable experience."

Toni, 43

sky as if you are greeting the sun. Your adominal muscles are pulled in, and you feel strong and centered.

4. As you exhale deeply, raise your arms even higher, fingers reaching, reaching, welcoming the force of life. Then inhale deeply.

5. As you exhale, bring your arms back down to waist level, and reach behind you as far as you can. It's a gentle reach. Stretch, but don't strain, your shoulders and chest muscles. Continue to breathe, slowly, deeply, and in rhythm with your movement. Be thankful that life has given you another day.

6. Bring your arms back to your sides and shake out your hands to release the energy.

7. Repeat the sequence four times, stretching a little more each time.

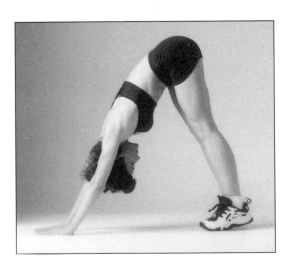

The second stretch is the Indian Goddess. As you do this stretch, feel your power, your absolute importance in the world. Acknowledge that you are accepted just the way you are.

1. Stand tall, with your legs a little wider than your hips. Your shoulders are down and relaxed, your neck long, and your eyes straight ahead.
2. As you inhale, slowly extend your arms away from your body, exhaling as you open your palms to the sky.
3. As you continue to breathe in and out in a deep, rhythmic manner, let your arms rise up to just below your shoulders, as if they were being carried by a gentle, invisible force.

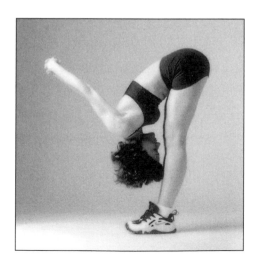

4. Feel your body become infused with power and light as you open your chest and stretch your wide arms back. You are offering yourself as a gift to the world.

5. Still breathing deeply, release your arms and let them swing lightly in front of your body—down and across, your left arm over your right arm. Swing back and repeat, right arm over your left arm. Do this twelve times in a graceful rhythm. You love yourself; you embrace yourself. Inhale on the open swing; exhale on the embracing motion.

Walk around for thirty seconds, taking long, deep breaths and shaking out your arms and hands. The final opening stretch, which is a static stretch, is designed for injury avoidance. It prepares your body to work. Do this stretch to prevent muscle strain and ligament tears. It will give you a greater range of motion in all of your joints.

1. Return to your initial standing position—feet slightly more than shoulder width apart, neck elongated, abs pulled in, eyes facing straight ahead.

2. Inhale. On the exhale, place your hands on your knees as you crouch slightly. Your head and back remain straight and still.

3. Continuing to breathe rhythmically, push your buttocks out and elongate your lower body. There is a nice unbroken line down the center of your back.

4. Crouch lower and place your hands on your shins, then crouch lower, bend your knees, drop your head down, and place your hands on your ankles. Keep breathing.

5. Bend more, place your hands on the fronts of your feet, and round your back.

6. Slowly straighten your legs (don't jerk them) while you keep your hands on the front of your feet, your head down, and your back rounded. Your buttocks rise slowly as you gently stretch your hamstrings. Hold. Count one, count two, count three, and slowly bend your knees, returning to your crouched position.

7. Repeat six times, breathing steadily in and out.

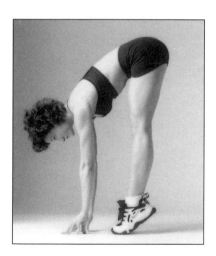

Workout: Fifteen to Twenty Minutes

Now you're ready to work. In this session, you're going to practice two exercises from the Determination and Integrity sections. They are:

Push-up

Lunge

Follow the directions previously outlined for each of these exercises. Your focus should be maintaining the proper form, identifying the muscles that are being worked, and learning to breathe through each motion. If you have trouble, check the DIVA Secrets and DIVA Troubleshooter sections. And always go back and check each aspect of your form. You can trust the exercises to do what they are supposed to do as long as you are in the correct position.

Perform each exercise ten times. Rest in between if you need to. Don't worry about mastering the exercise or criticizing yourself for not being perfect right away. Maintain the mentality of a beginner: curious and open to learning something new. It's important to practice each exercise and understand what's happening. Make sure you can say the instructions to yourself before you start doing repetitions.

After you have performed the exercises, walk around for a minute or so, shaking out your limbs and cooling down. Take a drink of water. Get your mat for the final stretch.

Stretch: Five to Seven Minutes

I think of the stretches at the end of a workout as the Meditation Stretches. The mood is quiet and reflective. These stretches beckon you to get completely inside yourself. Close off all the busy thoughts of the day. Give yourself over to the spirit of calm. At this moment, everything about your life is perfect. There are no worries. No past, no future. Just now.

1. Lie down on your back. As you inhale and exhale continually, lift your buttocks off the floor very slightly and then set them down a little further. You'll feel your lower back stretching and elongating.

2. Continue your breathing rhythm as you slowly bend your knees and bring your legs back toward your chest. Hold them lightly across your knees with your hands and stretch.

3. Release your right leg and gently slide it back down to the floor—not straight, but comfortably bent. Hold your left knee with both hands and stretch it back firmly and gently. The motion is smooth and natural.

4. Now, straighten your left leg above you, with the bottom of your foot facing the sky, your hands holding you beneath the knee. Hold for a moment, then flex your foot. Relax, then point your toes. Flex, point, flex, point . . . repeat four times.

5. Bend your knee and bring your leg down to your chest. Stretch it once more, then slide it back to the floor and bring your right leg up. Repeat the process with your right leg, then bring it down.

6. Take two or three deep breaths, and when you are ready, sit up.

7. Sit straight and tall, your neck elongated, your navel pulled. While breathing deeply in and out, slowly extend your legs outward in front of you in a straddle position—just until you feel a pulling in your groin muscles. (This

shouldn't be a severe or painful pulling. Don't try to stretch too wide at first.) Hold and breathe. Then release back by bringing your legs in just a bit until you don't feel the pulling. Open your legs out again, and hold.

8. Bring your arms down between your legs as you exhale. Let your torso come forward—slowly, not flopping—and keep your neck relaxed and head up as you bring your chest toward the floor. Try to feel your back elongating as you come forward. (Resist the tendency to bounce.) Hold the stretch for as long as you comfortably can, breathing deeply, then gently come back up to a sitting position, taking a final deep breath.

9. With your legs still open, stretch your torso toward the left, and place both arms over the left leg. Walk your hands down your leg as far as you can; try to reach your ankle or foot. Hold the position and continue breathing lightly. Then return to the center and take a nice, rewarding breath before you repeat the stretch on the other side. Make sure you keep the opposite hip down and the opposite leg on the floor.

10. Repeat each side three or four times, then stretch toward the center, torso over, arms leading, chest toward the floor. Then slowly roll back up, pulling your navel in and straightening your back from the bottom up, vertebra by vertebra.

11. Roll over onto your stomach. Bring your knees under you and raise up on all fours. Raise your head and slide your weight back into a crouch. Hold and breathe.

Now you're ready to live the rest of your day, empowered mentally, physically, and spiritually.

DIVA Troubleshooter

"True hope is swift and flies with swallow's wings."

Shakespeare

• **Why do you stretch at the end of the workout? Aren't you pretty well stretched by then?**

Stretching after exercising is part of your cooling down process. Mentally, you are preparing to return to the world. Physically, you are reassuring yourself that everything is in working order. A good stretch and cool-down routine goes a long way toward short-circuiting any potential muscle pain. It does that by helping to rid your body of lactic acid levels, which build up during exercise, and other metabolic wastes. The ending stretch also helps your heart rate return to normal and prevents the pooling of blood in your lower extremeties caused by a sudden cessation of exercise.

• **How do you know how far to stretch? What does it feel like when you've gone too far?**

Stretching is a different experience for every woman, depending on your body type, weight, level of conditioning, age, and mind-set. By mind-set I mean the ability to patiently put yourself through a series of movements that increase your flexibility and range of motion in all of your movable joints. While you're doing this, you must constantly focus on what you are experiencing, or you might injure yourself. It's normal to feel a pulling in your muscles; that's what stretching is all about. It's not normal to feel sharp, sudden pain or agonizing cramps in your arms, legs, or torso. That means you're aggravating the very areas you want to help. Know the difference between discomfort and pain. Discomfort usually ends when you release the area being stretched. Pain, however, is a specific, sharp ache, a localized sensation.

• Are there people who shouldn't stretch?

No matter your age, weight, or physical condition, every woman can benefit from a careful and systematic course of stretching. Your flexibility can be increased at any age. All it takes is the will to do it, and the patience to realize that the discomfort of going through it doesn't last forever, but the results *will*.

PART 3

THE
DIVA
LIFE

10

IT'S YOUR LIFE

Whenever a woman says to me, "I don't have time to exercise," I ask her, "Do you have time to eat?"

"Yes."

"Do you have time to sleep?"

"Yes."

"Do you have time to go to work?"

"Yes."

"Do you have time to . . ."

She'll usually stop me at this point. "I know what you're getting at," she'll say. "But I *have* to eat and sleep. I *have* to go to work. I don't have to exercise."

I guess that's the problem with some women's attitudes about exercise. Too many women see fitness as a supcrimposed grind instead of a natural extension of living, breathing, and moving. We all have a physiological memory of the time when women didn't need to exercise because life itself was an exercise. The labor-intensive lives that people lived prior to this cushy century made being in a state of fitness as important as getting up in the morning. There was no maybe about it.

In this section, we're going to talk about *life*. That means using your strength and fitness to empower you in everything. It's a great satisfaction to reach the point where your entire being—body, mind, and spirit—is operating in sync. That's what can happen when you live the DIVA life.

This section includes all of the elements you'll need to put the DIVA System into daily practice. It includes:

The Four Progressions (from easy to hard)
Food—a DIVA's best friend (really!)
The DIVA Journal (your vital record)

The system as I've outlined it here takes one year. But the time frame isn't what's important. Feel free to move at your own pace. Just don't skip any steps. You'll only be rushing to get nowhere. This is a life system, not an overnight sensation. It's got to live in your bones.

If the mention of doing this for a whole year makes you anxious, just ask yourself this question: What would you be doing with that year if not this? And what better way to spend a year . . . a decade . . . or the rest of your life?

Besides, the DIVA System has built-in features and flexibility that will keep you interested as you progress. There's nothing boring about this. Every step is a fresh challenge and a fresh victory.

A Word About Setting Goals

More than any other factor, I find that my students get into the most trouble because of the way they set their goals. People think that the definition of a goal is *anything in the world you want.* That's really not the definition. For example, if your goal is, "To grow four inches taller in four months," that would be laughable. Everyone knows our height is a given. You can't grow taller. So I'm going to suggest some parameters for your goal setting: Your goals need to be realistic, total, and flexible.

By *realistic,* I mean setting goals for your fitness level as well as your life that are achievable and personal. Pay attention to your own style and level. Learn to know your body and what it can do. Don't pattern yourself after others. Rather, use the input from others as a framework from which to create your own pattern.

By *total,* I mean refusing to see yourself as a collection of body parts. While one of your goals might be to tone your upper thighs, don't limit yourself to such rigid standards of success. Learn to measure your success not only by the number on the scale or tape measure, but also by the way you feel, your energy level, your competence, your understanding of the process, and your growing self-esteem.

By *flexible,* I mean giving yourself a break. Let yourself be a beginner. Use your failures as lessons. If you fall short of your goals one month, investigate the reasons why and adapt your pattern. You won't really know what works for you until you start moving.

This chart might help you discern the areas where you'll be setting goals. Add your own, too. This is the space for broad goals. The second sheet breaks the goals down into a three-month segment.

DIVA GOALS
Worksheet One

Goals	Three Months	Six Months	Nine Months	One Year
Fitness				
Self-image				
Nutrition				
Relationships				
Self-motivation				
Career				
Space				
Health				

DIVA GOALS
Worksheet Two

Three-Month Goal	The Eight Specific Steps I'll Take
Fitness	
Self-image	
Nutrition	
Relationships	
Self-motivation	
Career	
Space	
Health	

Never forget that living as a DIVA means being proud to be you. During this year, you have permission to focus on your personal goals and needs. Be self-involved, if only for that one hour. Remind yourself every day that the most reliable sign of your success is that you're doing it.

How to Use Your Journal

Your daily journal is an integral part of this system. It's far more than an objective record of what you do. It represents your unique journey. No one else is like you. Your journal is the place you roam freely to share your commitments, actions, successes, and struggles.

I learned the importance of the journal through experience with my students. I used to give each person a small exercise log to keep a record of what they did. Over time, I noticed that people were using the logs for more than just record keeping. They were writing about their experiences. They were recording what they ate every day. As I took their lead and began designing more complete journals for my students, I found that they were one of the best motivational tools I had ever known.

Your journal connects your mind, body, and spirit to the process. There are four elements in the journal:

1. PROGRESSION INFORMATION

This is the place where you write down where you are and what your long- and short-term goals are. Start by taking your measurements, but *do not* weigh yourself. Measurements are a more reliable standard. Don't make judgments; just write down the information. As you start working, you'll learn that the number on the scale is practically meaningless. Your measurements are a much more accurate guide to your level of strength and results.

Next, write your commitment to yourself. For example: "I will spend X hours every week practicing the exercises. I promise not to be too hard on myself and to be proud that I'm doing the work." The commitment is a personal thing. Give some thought to the barriers that have held you back in the past and how you're going to make an effort to overcome them.

Finally, write down your goals for a year and your goals for three months. Remember to be realistic, total, and flexible.

2. TRAINING LOG

The training log is the place you keep track of your workouts—right down to the number of repetitions, the duration, what you struggle with, and what your mood is while you're working. I urge my clients to be very specific here. It's one of the best ways to keep a record of your achievement. You can watch yourself move from awkwardness to competence, from five minutes to ten minutes, from twelve reps to twenty-four. When a student gets discouraged and complains to me that she doesn't feel like she's making progress, the first thing I do is have her review her training log. It's the written evidence of her progress.

3. FOOD DIARY

I don't encourage people to start focusing on food until Progression Two. That's because I don't want to make becoming a DIVA about that same old food issue that many women raise. I want you to feel your body and understand how it works before you start deciding how to best fuel it.

When you do begin using the food diary, it will help you learn what, when, and how much you eat. Believe it or not, most people aren't that aware of their daily diet. Over time, the food diary will serve as a more integral part of your daily life. You'll begin to recognize the relationship between what you eat and how you feel, and how you *perform* in your workouts.

As an aid to beginners, the food diary includes some basic suggestions about foods to eat. Notice that the focus is on healthy, fresh foods, not processed foods.

4. DIVA LIFE

This is the place where you talk to yourself about how you're doing, work out the difficulties you're having at work or with relationships, and reflect about how every piece of your life is linked to every other piece.

11

THE FOUR PROGRESSIONS OF THE DIVA SYSTEM

Progression One: Learning

Progression Two: Knowledge in action

Progression Three: Integration

Progression Four: Living it

PROGRESSION ONE: LEARNING

Progression One is the period of being a beginner: learning the exercises, learning them in combination, feeling your body, getting to know yourself.

Focus
- Creating a consistent routine
- Practicing and understanding the basic exercise techniques
- Gaining minimum strength
- Developing confidence that "Yes, I can do it."
- Learning realistic goal setting

CONCENTRATE ON . . .	DON'T WORRY ABOUT . . .
• learning the precise techniques	• Getting it right
• getting to know your body	• Seeing visible results
• believing you can do it	• Dieting
• sticking with it	• Feeling impatient to move on
• making a record in your journal	

Time Frame
Three months, plus or minus

If you've started to get the DIVA concept, you'll realize that every individual is unique, so I'm not going to say, "Progression One lasts three months—period!" For you, it may last two months, or it may last four. Just keep doing it until you're ready to move on.

The Workout Menu

Since the DIVA System is all about choice, Progression One gives you a workout menu with six combinations. Mix and match these combinations plus an aerobic activity throughout the three months. This method allows extra time for those exercises that are especially challenging for you. Total workout time should not exceed 45 minutes. The goal is to get as much done as efficiently as possible. As a beginner, you may take more time, but that should lessen as you become more efficient. Before you start, go back and review the workout routine in Aspiration. And a word of caution: Don't practice the jumps until you've mastered the squat and step-up.

The following are the six combinations on the Progression One Workout Menu.

WORKOUT MENU

Total Workout Time: 40-45 minutes

A TOTAL BODY CONCENTRATION

Aerobic warm-up

Stretch

Four sets of five push-ups

Two sets of ten squats
Three sets of ten basic abdominals
Cool down, stretch

B TOTAL BODY CONCENTRATION
Aerobic warm-up
Stretch
Two sets of five shoulder presses
Ten reps vertical jumps
Three sets of ten basic abdominals
Cool down, stretch

C UPPER BODY CONCENTRATION
Aerobic warm-up
Stretch
Two sets of ten dumbbell rows on each arm
Three sets of ten basic abdominals
Cool down, stretch

D LOWER BODY CONCENTRATION
Aerobic warm-up
Stretch
Two sets of ten lunges on each leg
Three sets of ten squats
Three sets of ten basic abdominals
Cool down, stretch

E LOWER BODY CONCENTRATION

Aerobic warm-up

Stretch

Three sets of ten stiff-legged dead lifts

Two sets of ten vertical jumps

Three sets of ten basic abdominals

Cool down, stretch

F UPPER BODY CONCENTRATION

Aerobic warm-up

Stretch

Two sets of ten side-to-side jumps

Three sets of ten push-ups

Three sets of ten basic abdominals

Cool down, stretch

AEROBIC ACTIVITY

Twice a week, choose an aerobic activity (see aerobic section in Vitality). Your aerobic activity should be designed as follows:

Warm-up

Stretch

Aerobic activity (work up to twenty minutes)

Cool down

Stretch

Total time: 30 minutes

Sample: One month

This sample is based on three workouts and two aerobic activities per week. Adapt it according to your need and ability. For example, an alternative might be two workouts and one aerobic activity or two workouts and two aerobic activities. You can also work on the combinations that suit your level. For example, you might spend one week (or three workouts) learning the A combination. It's up to you. The only guideline is that you do some aerobic activity every week and that you learn each exercise before you move on to Progression Two.

	M	T	W	TH	F	S	S
1.	A	aerobic	B	C	X	aerobic	X
2.	B	A	X	aerobic	C	X	aerobic
3.	D	aerobic	E	aerobic	X	F	X
4.	E	X	D	aerobic	X	F	aerobic

Are You Ready to Move on to Progression Two?

❑ Have you developed a routine that is at least three days a week and at least forty minutes each day?

❑ Do you have a physical and mental understanding of the techniques? Could you teach them to a friend?

❑ Do you feel stronger and more confident than you felt when you began to work?

Evaluate Your Ability to Comfortably and Correctly Perform the Exercises

These represent the minimum level of competency required to move on to Progression Two.

❑ I can perform at least ten bent-leg push-ups without resting.

❑ I can perform at least five straight-leg push-ups without resting.

❑ I automatically close my rib cage hinge every time I do crunches.

❑ I can perform at least twelve shoulder presses, seated or standing, without resting.

❑ I don't feel any strain or tension in my neck and shoulders when I do a shoulder press.

❑ I can do at least eight dumbbell rows on each side without resting.

❑ My lower back doesn't feel any strain when I do dumbbell rows.

❑ I can perform at least twelve lunges, alternating left and right legs, without resting.

❑ I feel my shoulders automatically relaxing and don't have any tendency to hunch them up.

❑ When I do a lunge, I don't lean to the side or lose my balance.

❑ I can feel my abdominal muscles working when I do ab exercises.

❑ I can feel my abdominal muscles working when I do every exercise.

❑ During abdominals, my lower back is pushed into the floor and my breathing is deep and rhythmic.

❑ I can perform ten steady cable balance reps on each leg without wavering.

❑ I bend from the hips, not the waist, to do dead lifts.

❑ Step-ups don't throw me out of balance. I can do fifteen in a row without stopping.

❑ I don't feel squats in my knees or in my lower back. I can do fifteen without stopping.

❑ I've conquered my fear of jumping.

❑ I am able to comfortably do more than twenty minutes of aerobic exercise in my heart rate zone.

❑ I don't skimp with warm-ups or stretches when I do my workouts.

❑ I can describe at least five ways the workouts have helped me in everyday life.

If Ten to Fifteen Boxes Are Not Checked

- Return to Progression One for one month.
- Study your results and find the areas in which you have the most trouble: strength? stability? flexibility? aerobic duration? Find combinations on the menu that will give you intensive practice in those areas.
- If your problem is consistency, go back to your goals and study your journal entries. What's stopping you?
- Don't give up. Work it through and reevaluate in one month.

If Ten Boxes Are Not Checked

Return to Progression One for two weeks.

Design your own combinations that will allow you to focus on the areas of weakness. (But be sure to incorporate aerobics.)

If Every Box Is Checked

Move on to Progression Two.

STRAIGHT TALK ABOUT SUCCESS AND FAILURE

If you're in that box that says, "Go back and try again," I know how you're feeling. The reason I know is that it's just human nature to think you're incompetent when it takes you longer than average to master something, or to think you've failed when everyone is moving to the head of the class except you. This is that dangerous moment when the little voice of doubt starts whispering its discouraging mantra in your ear: "I knew I couldn't do it. I tried, and look what happened. I'm just not athletic. What's the point of this? It's too hard. I feel stupid." *But wait!* I think you're forgetting something. You're forgetting that you're a DIVA. You measure success and failure by different standards than others. Success does not mean you've met someone else's arbitrary standards (and let's face it; the three-month time frame is arbitrary, because I can't know what works for you as an individual. The important thing is, are you meeting your own standards? If you're not, why not? Are you setting unrealistic goals? Are you allowing self-doubt to paralyze you? Are you having trouble believing in yourself? Write about it in your journal. Once you express it, you've already cleared the way and you're moving ahead.

PROGRESSION TWO: KNOWLEDGE IN ACTION

When you reach Progression Two, you will be ready to start working on nutrition. I will give you some ideas about how you can retrain your taste buds away from processed foods and toward fresh foods. You'll find that it feels natural and right to eat fresh foods as your changing body will crave them more and more.

Focus

- Moving from the image of *learning* to the image of *knowing*
- Adding the nutrition element
- Graduating to more advanced movements
- Increasing your speed and confidence
- Finding the evidence of success

CONCENTRATE ON . . .	DON'T WORRY ABOUT . . .
• Owning the workout	• Struggling with new steps
• Appreciating your results	• Scales and tape measures
• Finding power in daily life	• Comparing yourself to others
• Feeling the food/energy connection in your body	• Eating a perfect diet (as defined by others)

Time Frame

Three months. It depends on your pace. Don't skip any steps.

The Workout Menu

Progression Two gives you a workout menu with six combinations. Mix and match them any way that feels right. In addition, add time to your aerobic workouts. For instructions about beginning the food work, refer to chapter 12.

The following are the six combinations on the Progression Two Workout Menu.

WORKOUT MENU

Total Workout Time: 40–45 minutes

A LOWER BODY CONCENTRATION

Aerobic warm-up—20 minutes
Stretch
Three sets of ten push-ups
Three sets of fifteen stiff-legged dead lifts
Three sets of fifteen squats
Three sets of fifteen vertical jumps
Four to six sets of fifteen abdominal crunches
Cool-down, stretch

B LOWER BODY CONCENTRATION

Aerobic warm-up—20 minutes

Stretch

Three sets of ten shoulder presses

Three sets of fifteen cable balances on each leg

Three sets of fifteen step-ups on each leg

Three sets of fifteen side-to-side jumps

Four to six sets of fifteen abdominal crunches

Cool down, stretch

C UPPER BODY CONCENTRATION

Aerobic warm-up—20 minutes

Stretch

Three sets of ten shoulder presses

Three sets of ten push-ups

Three sets of ten dumbbell rows on each side

Three sets of fifteen stiff-legged dead lifts

Three to five sets of fifteen abdominal crunches

Cool down, stretch

D LOWER BODY CONCENTRATION

Aerobic warm-up—20 minutes

Stretch

Three sets of fifteen lunges on each leg

Three sets of fifteen cable balances on each leg

Three sets of fifteen step-ups on each leg

Three sets of fifteen squats

Two to three sets each: vertical jumps, side-to-side jumps,
    front and back jumps

Three to five sets abdominal crunches

Cool-down, stretch

E TOTAL BODY CONCENTRATION

Aerobic warm-up—20 minutes

Stretch

Two sets each: vertical jumps, side-to-side jumps, back-
front jumps, rotating

Three sets of dumbbell rows on each side

Two sets of fifteen consecutive push-ups

Four to six sets of ten abdominal crunches

Cool down, stretch

F TOTAL BODY CONCENTRATION

Aerobic warm-up—20 minutes

Stretch

Two sets of fifteen cable balances on each leg

Two sets of twenty-five step-ups on each leg without stopping

Two sets of fifteen stiff-legged dead lifts without stopping

Two sets of fifteen straight-legged push-ups without stopping

Four to eight sets of ten abdominal crunches

Cool down, stretch

AEROBIC ACTIVITY

Push yourself harder. Add five minutes of aerobic activity to your warm-up. Try to increase your heart rate during exercise. Maintain the routine of warm-ups, cool-downs, and stretches.

Sample: One month

This sample is based on three workouts and two aerobic activities per week. Adapt it according to your need and ability. During Progression Two, you won't be changing the number of days; you'll be changing the length and intensity of your work.

	M	T	W	TH	F	S	S
1.	A	aerobic	B	C	X	aerobic	X
2.	B	A	X	aerobic	C	X	aerobic
3.	D	aerobic	E	aerobic	X	F	X
4.	E	X	D	aerobic	X	F	aerobic

Are You Ready to Move on to Progression Three?

❑ Have you been consistent in working at least three days a week, and have you increased your workouts and aerobic activity by about five minutes each time?

❑ Have you done the work in your food diary and made the connection between food and fuel for working?

❑ Have you seen small examples every week of success that you can point to?

Evaluate Your Ability to Comfortably and Correctly Do the Work

These represent the minimum level of competency required to move on to Progression Three.

- ❏ I can work for forty minutes at a time without feeling overly strained or sore.
- ❏ I've increased my aerobic workouts by fifteen to twenty minutes, three times a week.
- ❏ I've measured an increase in my maximum heart rate during aerobic exercise.
- ❏ I am writing in my journal every day.
- ❏ I have noticed positive changes in my life—beyond fitness. I can point to specific ways this work has improved my job, attitudes, relationships, etc.
- ❏ I feel confident that I know and own the individual exercises.
- ❏ I have kept a food diary.
- ❏ I have made positive changes in my diet that directly relate to this work.
- ❏ I have started to see measurable signs of improvement— in my weight, posture, strength, flexibility, agility, or other.

If Many Boxes Are Not Checked

Return to Progression Two for one month.

Study your results and find the areas in which you have the most trouble: strength? stability? flexibility? aerobic duration? food? consistency? commitment? life improvements? fitness improvements?

If your problem is consistency, go back to your goals and study your journal entries. What's stopping you?

Don't give up. Work it through and reevaluate in one month.

If Just a Few Boxes Are Not Checked

Return to Progression Two for two weeks.

Design your own combinations that will allow you to focus on the areas of weakness. (But be sure to incorporate aerobics.)

If Every Box Is Checked

Move on to Progression Three.

PROGRESSION THREE: INTEGRATION

As you begin to gain strength and confidence, your goals will change. The work will become more skill-based. You'll be comfortable with the routine; the emphasis will be on doing more. This is probably the most difficult period of the program—what is sometimes called hitting a plateau. To keep you inspired, awake, and eager to work, I'll vary the workouts during this phase, incorporating aerobics and weight work.

Focus

- Maintaining consistency
- Developing motion skills
- Increasing strength and endurance
- Becoming more efficient by reducing the time of sessions

CONCENTRATE ON . . .

- Staying focused

- Pushing yourself to do more in less time
- Feeling the intensity
- Being in the work
- Taking the work out with you

DON'T WORRY ABOUT . . .

- Occasional feelings of lethargy

- Doing too much
- Tomorrow . . . just do it today

Time Frame

Three months. Don't skimp on this progression. It's the real groundwork for your life plan.

The Workout Menu

There are six combinations in Progression Three, each one very demanding in a different way. If you find that these workouts are too hard, go back to Progression Two for a couple of weeks. You'll probably need to concentrate on increasing your weights and number of sets to make sure you're prepared to move on. Remember: Each Progression builds upon the previous one. The following are the six combinations on the Progression Three Menu.

WORKOUT MENU

A TOTAL BODY CONCENTRATION

Aerobic warm-up

Stretch

Twenty to thirty minutes of aerobics

Three sets of ten straight-legged push-ups

Three sets of twenty stiff-legged deadlifts—with added
  weight

Three sets of twenty squats, holding bar or dumbells

Four sets of fifteen basic abdominal crunches

Four sets of fifteen advanced abdominal crunches

Cool-down, stretch

Work for thirty to forty minutes total.

B LOWER BODY CONCENTRATION

Aerobic warm-up

Stretch

Three sets of twenty cable balances on each leg

Three sets of ten squats with weight bar

Ten sets of three-jump combination: vertical, side-to-side,
   front-back, without stopping

Five sets of ten basic abdominal crunches

Four sets of ten advanced abdominal crunches

Cool-down, stretch

Work for twenty-thirty minutes total.

C UPPER BODY CONCENTRATION

Aerobic warm-up

Stretch

Twenty to thirty minutes of aerobics

Three sets of ten standing shoulder presses—add weight

Three sets of ten dumbbell rows on each side—add
   weight

Three sets of ten lunges on each side—add weight

Five to ten sets of ten basic or advanced abdominals

Cool-down, stretch

Work for thirty to forty-five minutes total.

D TOTAL BODY CONCENTRATION

Aerobic warm-up

Stretch

One set of ten straight-legged push-ups

Two sets of ten standing shoulder presses with added
   weight

Two sets of ten dumbell rows on each side with added
weight
Two sets of ten lunges on each leg with added weight
Two sets of ten step-ups on each leg with added weight
Two sets of ten squats with added weight
Six to twelve sets of ten advanced abdominals
Cool-down, stretch
Work for twenty to thirty minutes total.

E UPPER BODY CONCENTRATION

Aerobic warm-up
Stretch
Twenty to thirty minutes of aerobics
Upper Body Only
Forty consecutive push-ups (knee and straight-leg com-
bos)
Two sets of twenty shoulder presses
Two sets of twenty dumbbell rows on each side
Two sets of twenty stiff-legged dead lifts
Four sets of fifteen advanced abdominals
Cool down, stretch
Work for thirty to forty minutes total.

F LOWER BODY CONCENTRATION

Aerobic warm-up
Stretch
Lower Body Only
Two to three sets of twenty alternating lunges on each leg
Two sets of twenty cable balances on each leg
Two to three sets of thirty step-ups on each leg

Two sets of fifteen squats

Three sets of ten side-to-side jumps

Four sets of twenty abdominals

Cool-down, stretch

Work for thirty to forty-five minutes total.

AEROBIC ACTIVITY

Progression Three aerobic exercises are incorporated into the workouts. This is the integration that occurs as you advance. It's a powerful way to feel your body in motion—in every respect: muscle-by-muscle and the whole body. You might want to push yourself to add one full aerobic activity day per week, in addition to your four scheduled workouts. Remember to stay within your time frame!

Sample: One month

This sample is based on four full workouts a week, incorporating aerobic activity. You can also add another day and just do an aerobic activity. Be sure you're ready for this advanced work before you start. Choose from six combinations.

	M	T	W	TH	F	S	S
1.	A	B	X	C	X	X	D
2.	C	X	A	X	C	X	E
3.	D	aerobic	F	X	A	B	C
4.	X	E	D	aerobic	F	aerobic	X

Are You Ready to Move on to Progression Four?

❏ Have you been consistent in working at least four days a week, incorporating workouts and aerobics? Have you added a day of aerobics during some weeks?

❏ Have you done the work in your food diary and made significant changes in your diet for which you have seen tangible results?

❏ Are you continuing to see examples every week of success that you can point to?

❏ Have you been getting more work done in the same amount or less time?

❏ Have you been adding weight and increasing your reps day by day?

Evaluate Where You Stand at the End of Nine Months

Progression Four is an entirely new physical and mental challenge.

These statements must be true before you can move on to Progression Four.

❏ I am comfortable working on my own or with others.

❏ I am self-motivated and no longer fear that I'll give up.

❏ I can mix aerobic and strength exercises without overtiring myself. In fact, it feels exhilarating.

❏ I know when to add weight to any exercise, or increase the number of reps.

❏ I am definitely stronger.

❏ I understand the relationship between what I eat and my energy level.

❑ My body looks different: stronger, leaner, more erect, better toned, etc. These are visible changes I can see in a mirror.

❑ I'm not obsessed about my body's weight and shape. I see that my body is finding its own perfect balance.

❑ I no longer fear food.

❑ I have a new sense of my power in the world.

❑ I'm ready for new challenges.

If Many Boxes Are Not Checked

- Return to Progression Three for one month.
- Study your results and find the areas in which you have the most trouble: strength? stability? flexibility? aerobic duration? food? consistency? commitment? life improvements? fitness improvements?
- If your problem is consistency, go back to your goals and study your journal entries. What's stopping you?
- This is a critical juncture. If you're not ready to create your own routine, don't push it.

If Just a Few Boxes Are Not Checked

Return to Progression Three for two weeks until you have more confidence.

If Every Box Is Checked

Move on to Progression Four.

PROGRESSION FOUR: LIVING IT

The first nine months have been focused on creating a pattern—the habit of moving and being fully engaged in your body and mind. Now, you really begin to *live* what you've learned. My primary goal as a teacher and motivator is to help you do this work on your own and adapt it to your lifestyle and personal goals. That's what the final segment of this year will involve. You're going to leave the nest.

Focus

- Living it—being more flexible and spontaneous
- Discovering how far you can push yourself
- Internalizing that exercise is as fundamental as brushing your teeth
- Becoming your own trainer
- Knowing in your bones that you're a DIVA

Time Frame

Anywhere from three months to the rest of your life.

Your Workout Challenge

There is no menu for Progression Four—at least, not until you create one. In this stage, everything you do will be generated by you. It's your way of putting a personal stamp on it—to own the work as yours. There are two elements:

1. Create your own workout.
2. Choose a sport, or a new activity.

CREATE YOUR OWN WORKOUT

How are you going to be certain that all your muscles are being worked on a regular basis and that you're getting sufficient aerobic exercise? Go back and review: Determination, Integrity, Vitality, and Aspiration. For each exercise, ask yourself:

• How can I make this exercise more advanced?
• How can I do this exercise faster, without compromising form and technique?
• Which exercises can I combine for speed and agility?
• Will I be challenged by doing a circuit of all the DIVA exercises without resting?
• How can I incorporate aerobic activity with weight?
• How can I intensify my work in the areas where I still have the most trouble?

Now, create six combinations or specialized workouts of your own, placing a time frame on each set. (Actually, you can create more than six if you want to.) Always include your warm-up, stretches, and cool-down, then vary the order in which you perform the exercises. When you've designed your workouts, write them in the spaces. Make sure there is a balance of upper- and lower-body exercises, and you don't neglect either your upper or lower body. If you do upper-body one day, do lower-body the next day. If you work your entire body, be sure you rest the next day—or just do aerobics or stretching.

A
    Warm-up
    Stretch

    Cool down, stretch

B
    Warm-up
    Stretch

    Cool down, stretch

C
    Warm-up
    Stretch

    Cool down, stretch

D

Warm-up
Stretch

Cool down, stretch

E

Warm-up
Stretch

Cool down, stretch

F

Warm-up
Stretch

Cool down, stretch

CHOOSE A SPORT OR A NEW ACTIVITY

Are you scratching your head and thinking, "A *sport?* I'm not a sports type." Don't be intimidated. I don't mean you should go out and start playing hockey or competitive volleyball—unless, of course, you *want* to. A sport is something you decide to do because it's fun. If you've never played a sport before, you may not even know where to begin.

I'll give you a hint. Think way back to a time when you were eight or nine years old, before people started saying, "Girls don't do that," or, "Girls don't act that way." Then you felt totally free to love whatever you loved. What kind of physical activity did you enjoy? Was it solitary or in a group? Did it involve strength, speed, coordination—or all of them? What did you love about it? Recapture that feeling today. Decide to pick up where you left off.

You may be amazed to discover that you can do things you wouldn't have thought would be in your reach. One of my students, a forty-year-old woman who had never exercised regularly as an adult and had always been embarrassed about being clumsy, announced after a year of work that she was interested in taking up cross-country skiing. Her eyes were shining when she told me this. After forty years, she had discovered a wonderful new side to herself that had been dormant for many years.

Another student remembered how much she had loved to roller skate when she was a child. She would skate for hours without stopping. She described her pleasure at the feeling of speed and energy, the way the wind whipped at her cheeks, and the daring involved in going down hills. I asked if she would like to recapture that pleasure by learning to Rollerblade. At first, she said, "No, I can't. It's too dangerous." I reminded her that she had loved that feeling when she was young, and, besides, it's not really so dangerous if you learn it correctly. And with the right equipment, no skinned elbows and knees, either (something else she remembered from her childhood). Finally, she agreed, and she's glad she did. It's been a big breakthrough for her to see that exercise and fitness can be found in play. What a bargain!

Even if you don't have any fond childhood memories of physical play, you probably have a secret wish about being able to do something that you've always felt you couldn't do. I once had a student in her mid-thirties who was embarrassed to admit that she couldn't swim. She'd never learned as a child, and she thought it would be too humiliating to learn as an adult. Meanwhile, she was filled with envy every time she went to a pool or beach and saw how much fun people were having in the water. I urged her to find a pool where private lessons were given. Within a few months, she knew how to swim. Now, you can't keep her out of the water.

A similar thing happened with an eighteen-year-old girl who didn't know how to ride a bike. That may seem hard to imagine. Most people learn to ride bikes when they're kids. But she lived in the city, and her parents thought biking was too dangerous on the mean streets, so she never learned. I took her to Central Park, rented a bike, and taught her. It was a simple exercise, but what a thrill for her.

As the final step of learning to be a DIVA in action, find that dream of physical competence deep down inside, and go after it. Fitness is only a fraction of what you'll gain.

12

As you begin to explore the relationship between food and the principles of DIVA, you will have to give up all of your old biases about eating. I know what those biases are. I've heard them stated a thousand times.

Food is temptation.

Food means being out of control.

Food means gaining weight.

Food means wanting things I can't have.

Food gets in the way of my success.

Food gives me comfort.

Food makes me guilty.

Food is the enemy.

I want to suggest to you that there's a whole new set of possibilities about what food can mean to you.

Food means energy.

Food means strength.

Food means having enough vitality to work.

Food means not getting tired before the end.

Food means not feeling weak.

Food means having what I need.

Food means nourishment.

Food means muscle.

Food means brainpower.

Food is my best friend.

The shift we're going to make, first in thinking and then in experience, is away from food as the bane of every woman's hips to food as the fuel that keeps the engine of your life moving. It may not be an easy change to make if you've been brainwashed about food all of your life, but once you get it, it will feel like a huge weight has been removed from the pit of your stomach. Imagine never having to *worry* about food again!

I ask you to have the patience to follow this system, even though the steps are slow and methodical. I assure you, it will be worth it to make your peace with nature's bounty.

Beginning with Progression Two, Keep a Food Diary Every Day

In the beginning, I won't ask you to change anything about your diet. Just eat the way you normally do, but keep track of what you eat. As you begin to develop an awareness of your body, you'll be able to evaluate how your diet is helping or getting in the way. You'll find the connection between what, when, and how much you eat and how you feel; for example, do you have energy, strength, endurance? As you learn to make the connection between food and movement, I'll help you start to make the adjustments in your diet that will complement your physical work.

In the beginning, the food diary helps you learn what, when, and how much you eat. Believe it or not, most people aren't that aware of their daily diet.

Over time, the food diary will serve as a more integral part of your daily life. You'll begin to recognize the relationship between what you eat and how you feel, move, and perform.

FIRST MONTH: AWARENESS
(REMEMBER: THIS PART SHOULD COORDINATE
WITH LEVEL 2)

WEEK ONE

Write down everything you eat (food and amount), when you eat it (the time on the clock), and where you are when you're eating. Don't judge. Just record.

WEEK TWO

In addition to recording what/when/where you eat, notice and write down how you feel right before you eat. Do you feel hungry, bored, restless, tired, upset, happy, neutral? Don't judge. Just record.

WEEK THREE

In addition to recording what/when/where you eat and how you feel before you eat, write down how you feel in the hours after you eat. Do you feel sluggish and tired, revved up and raring to go, unhappy, guilty, relaxed? Don't judge. Just record.

WEEK FOUR

In addition to continuing all of the observations from the first three weeks, notice the times you don't eat; for example, when you skip breakfast or lunch. Do you feel weak and hungry all morning? Do you find it harder to get going? Does not eating interfere wih your productivity? Do you find yourself overeating at night to compensate?

AT THE END OF WEEK FOUR, MAKE NOTES IN YOUR JOURNAL

What have you learned about the foods you eat? Are they primarily protein or carbohydrate? Are there any major food categories that are missing from your diet such as green vegetables, fish, dairy, etc.? What percentage of the food you eat is empty calories such as sugar, sodas, coffee, candy, snack foods?

What time of the day do you tend to eat the most food? The least? Do you plan your meals, or do you usually grab a snack or fast food when you're hungry? Do you try to put off eating for as long as you can? Does your schedule sometimes interfere with the times you'd prefer to be eating?

Where do you usually eat? At a table? Standing up? Munching on the street? In bed? How do you choose where you eat? It just happens? You plan it?

What did you discover about how you usually feel just before you eat? Do you eat because you're hungry? Because you've scheduled a meal? Because you know you need nourishment? Or do you sometimes eat because you're bored, depressed, or at loose ends? What relationship does your mood have to when and what you eat?

What did you discover about how you feel in the hours after you eat? Do you feel fueled for action? Do you feel sluggish and sleepy? Try to make a connection between what and when you eat and how it makes you feel.

What did you discover about your meal-skipping pattern? That you don't skip meals? That you often skip meals? What are the consequences of skipping meals? Do you feel extra hungry? Do you feel light-headed or sick? Do you overeat later to compensate?

SECOND MONTH: EXPERIMENTATION

WEEK FIVE
Based on your evaluation of the first month, make *one* change that you think will improve your energy, endurance, physical condition, or attitude. For example, if you discovered that skipping breakfast makes you feel tired in the morning, eat something every morning before you leave the house. If you found that eating on the run forced you to eat foods that were fatty and unhealthy, plan to carry a lunch. Write down the results of this change.

WEEK SIX
Make one more change, again based on your evaluation of the first month. Write down the results of this change.

WEEK SEVEN
Make a third change and write down the results.

WEEK EIGHT
Make a fourth change and write down the results.

AT THE END OF WEEK EIGHT, WRITE IN YOUR JOURNAL
What happened when you made each change? What did you learn about your relationship to food? What did you learn about food's relationship to the way your body works?

THIRD MONTH: LIVING WITH THE CHANGES

For the next month, continue to live with all four of the changes you made. Try them on to see how they feel. You may find that you're not sure how to integrate them. Here are some tips on making good nutrition choices:

1. Eat at least three meals a day, or four *small* meals.
2. Be sure to eat a *variety* of foods.
3. Forget about low fat, no fat products. They usually just substitute sugar, sodium or chemicals for fat.
4. Eat when you're hungry; stop when you're full.
5. Don't eat late at night. Consume most of your food when you are metabolically active.

What has changed about the way you eat?

What benefits have you noticed about making these changes?

How would you now state your motivation for change in your diet?

FOURTH MONTH: INTEGRATING FOOD WITH EXERCISE

During this month, pay special attention to your eating on the days that you exercise. Follow these guidelines:

- Never skip breakfast on a day that you're exercising.
- Experiment with foods to find the ones that give you more energy.
- Drink several glasses of water each day.
- On the days you exercise, eliminate the empty foods that don't add anything to your workout.

At the End of Week Twelve, Write in Your Journal

Did your consciousness about food make a difference in your energy, strength, or flexibility during your workout? If so, in what ways?

This is the step in your journey where you finally make the connection between the foods you put in your body and the way your body operates. This connection frees you at last from the fears that may have plagued you about food.

Living with Your Nutrition Plan

You have now spent four months experimenting and investigating how food relates to the circle of your life, in which everything is a part of the whole. If you've been following the DIVA System, you're beginning to experience a direct relationship between how you eat and how you live. I'm not going to give you food lists and portion sizes, because you don't need them. The best diet is the one that helps you do what you need to do and be what you need to be. I'll give you a hint, though: Real food is natural. If you have to squint to read the list of chemicals and additives, who needs it? The best foods for strength, energy, and health are those that are in their most natural state: Lean meat, fresh fish, fresh dairy, whole grains, and fresh vegetables and fruits. Eat as much as you need, but keep it simple, and get on with your life.

DIVA JOURNAL

*"Of my own spirit let me be
in sole though feeble mastery."*
Sara Teasdale

*NAME*_____

Progression One: Learning

Personal Evaluation

Date: _____

Age: _____

MEASUREMENTS:

Chest _____   Thigh _____

Waist _____   Calf _____

Hip _____   Arm _____

COMMITMENT:

During Progression One, I challenge myself to

_____

_____

_____

_____

_____

I-YEAR GOALS   3-MONTH GOALS

FITNESS   FITNESS

LIFE   LIFE

Progression Two: Knowledge in Action

Personal Evaluation

Date: _____

Age:_____

MEASUREMENTS:

    Chest _____   Thigh _____

    Waist _____   Calf _____

    Hip _____   Arm _____

COMMITMENT:

    During Progression Two, I challenge myself to

_____

_____

_____

_____

_____

1-YEAR GOALS	3-MONTH GOALS
FITNESS	FITNESS
LIFE	LIFE

Progression Three: Integration

Personal Evaluation

Date: _____

Age: _____

MEASUREMENTS:

    Chest _____   Thigh _____

    Waist _____   Calf _____

    Hip _____   Arm _____

COMMITMENT:

    During Progression Three, I challenge myself to

_____

_____

_____

_____

_____

1-YEAR GOALS	3-MONTH GOALS
FITNESS	FITNESS
LIFE	LIFE

Progression Four: Living It

Personal Evaluation

Date: _____
Age: _____

MEASUREMENTS:

Chest _____   Thigh _____

Waist _____   Calf _____

Hip _____   Arm _____

COMMITMENT:

During Progression Four, I challenge myself to

_____

_____

_____

_____

_____

1-YEAR GOALS	3-MONTH GOALS
FITNESS	FITNESS
LIFE	LIFE

DIVA Training Log

Date_____

Progression # _____

Time of Day_____

Combination # _____

Exercise	Weights	Reps	Level	Aerobic/ duration	Heart Rate (6 seconds × 10)	
_____	_____	_____	_____	_____	warm up	_____
_____	_____	_____	_____	_____	half way	_____
_____	_____	_____	_____	_____	end	_____
_____	_____	_____	_____	_____		

Today I learned:

Today I noticed these improvements:

Today I noticed these difficulties:

Today I experienced myself as a DIVA when:

DIVA Training Log

Date_____   Progression # _____

Time of Day_____   Combination # _____

Exercise	Weights	Reps	Level	Aerobic/ duration	Heart Rate (6 seconds × 10)	
_____	_____	_____	_____	_____	warm up	_____
_____	_____	_____	_____	_____	half way	_____
_____	_____	_____	_____	_____	end	_____
_____	_____	_____	_____	_____		

Today I learned:

Today I noticed these improvements:

Today I noticed these difficulties:

Today I experienced myself as a DIVA when:

DIVA Training Log

Date_____   Progression # _____

Time of Day_____   Combination # _____

Exercise	Weights	Reps	Level	Aerobic/ duration	Heart Rate (6 seconds × 10)	
_____	_____	_____	_____	_____	warm up	_____
_____	_____	_____	_____	_____	half way	_____
_____	_____	_____	_____	_____	end	_____
_____	_____	_____	_____	_____		

Today I learned:

Today I noticed these improvements:

Today I noticed these difficulties:

Today I experienced myself as a DIVA when:

DIVA Training Log

Date_____   Progression # _____

Time of Day_____   Combination # _____

Exercise	Weights	Reps	Level	Aerobic/ duration	Heart Rate (6 seconds × 10)	
_____	_____	_____	_____	_____	warm up	_____
_____	_____	_____	_____	_____	half way	_____
_____	_____	_____	_____	_____	end	_____
_____	_____	_____	_____	_____		

Today I learned:

Today I noticed these improvements:

Today I noticed these difficulties:

Today I experienced myself as a DIVA when:

DIVA Training Log

Date_____   Progression # _____

Time of Day_____   Combination # _____

Exercise	Weights	Reps	Level	Aerobic/ duration	Heart Rate (6 seconds × 10)	
_____	_____	_____	_____	_____	warm up	_____
_____	_____	_____	_____	_____	half way	_____
_____	_____	_____	_____	_____	end	_____
_____	_____	_____	_____	_____		

Today I learned:

Today I noticed these improvements:

Today I noticed these difficulties:

Today I experienced myself as a DIVA when:

DIVA Training Log

Date_____   Progression # _____

Time of Day_____   Combination # _____

Exercise	Weights	Reps	Level	Aerobic/ duration	Heart Rate (6 seconds × 10)	
_____	_____	_____	_____	_____	warm up	_____
_____	_____	_____	_____	_____	half way	_____
_____	_____	_____	_____	_____	end	_____
_____	_____	_____	_____	_____		

Today I learned:

Today I noticed these improvements:

Today I noticed these difficulties:

Today I experienced myself as a DIVA when:

DIVA Training Log

Date_____   Progression # _____

Time of Day_____   Combination # _____

Exercise	Weights	Reps	Level	Aerobic/ duration	Heart Rate (6 seconds × 10)	
_____	_____	_____	_____	_____	warm up	_____
_____	_____	_____	_____	_____	half way	_____
_____	_____	_____	_____	_____	end	_____
_____	_____	_____	_____	_____		

Today I learned:

Today I noticed these improvements:

Today I noticed these difficulties:

Today I experienced myself as a DIVA when:

DIVA Food Diary

Day _____   Date _____

	What I ate	Time	Place	How I Felt
Breakfast				
Lunch				
Dinner				
Snacks				

Comments:

My mood today was:

DIVA Food Diary

Day _____   Date _____

	What I ate	Time	Place	How I Felt
Breakfast				
Lunch				
Dinner				
Snacks				

Comments:

My mood today was:

DIVA Food Diary

Day _____   Date _____

	What I ate	Time	Place	How I Felt
Breakfast				
Lunch				
Dinner				
Snacks				

Comments:

My mood today was:

DIVA Food Diary

Day _____ Date _____

	What I ate	Time	Place	How I Felt
Breakfast				
Lunch				
Dinner				
Snacks				

Comments:

My mood today was:

DIVA Food Diary

Day _____   Date _____

	What I ate	Time	Place	How I Felt
Breakfast				
Lunch				
Dinner				
Snacks				

Comments:

My mood today was:

DIVA Food Diary

Day _____ Date _____

	What I ate	Time	Place	How I Felt
Breakfast				
Lunch				
Dinner				
Snacks				

Comments:

My mood today was:

DIVA Food Diary

Day _____   Date _____

	What I ate	Time	Place	How I Felt
Breakfast				
Lunch				
Dinner				
Snacks				

Comments:

My mood today was:

Life Work

My Private Reflections

Date_____   Time _____

_____

Date_____   Time _____

Life Work

My Private Reflections

Date_____   Time _____

_____

Date_____   Time _____

Life Work

My Private Reflections

Date_____   Time _____

_____

Date_____   Time _____

Life Work

My Private Reflections

Date_____   Time _____

_____

Date_____   Time _____

Life Work

My Private Reflections

Date_____   Time _____

_____

Date_____   Time _____

Life Work

My Private Reflections

Date_____   Time _____

_____

Date_____   Time _____

Life Work

My Private Reflections

Date_____   Time _____

_____

Date_____   Time _____